VITAMINS AND
CANCER PREVENTION

CONTEMPORARY ISSUES IN CLINICAL NUTRITION

Series Editor
Richard S. Rivlin, M.D.

Contemporary Issues in Clinical Nutrition, Volumes 1–7, were published by Churchill Livingstone, Inc.

VITAMINS AND CANCER PREVENTION

Editors

Stewart A. Laidlaw, Ph.D.
Division of Medical Oncology
UCLA Schools of Medicine and Public Health
Harbor-UCLA Medical Center
Torrance, California

Marian E. Swendseid, Ph.D.
Division of Nutrition Sciences
UCLA School of Public Health
Los Angeles, California

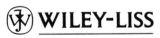 **WILEY-LISS**

A JOHN WILEY & SONS, INC., PUBLICATION
New York • Chichester • Brisbane • Toronto • Singapore

Address all Inquiries to the Publisher
Wiley-Liss, Inc., 41 East 11th Street, New York, NY 10003

Copyright © 1991 Wiley-Liss, Inc.

Printed in United States of America

While the authors, editors, and publisher believe that drug selection and dosage and the specifications and usage of equipment and devices, as set forth in this book, are in accord with current recommendations and practice at the time of publication, they accept no legal responsibility for any errors or omissions, and make no warranty, express or implied, with respect to material contained herein. In view of ongoing research, equipment modifications, changes in governmental regulations and the constant flow of information relating to drug therapy, drug reactions and the use of equipment and devices, the reader is urged to review and evaluate the information provided in the package insert or instructions for each drug, piece of equipment or device for, among other things, any changes in the instructions or indications of dosage or usage and for added warnings and precautions.

Library of Congress Cataloging-in-Publication Data

Vitamins and cancer prevention / editors, Stewart A. Laidlaw, Marian
    E. Swendseid
        p.   cm. — (Contemporary issues in clinical nutrition ; v. 14)
    "Proceedings of the Gladys Emerson-UCLA Clinical Nutrition
Research Unit Symposium, March 2–3, 1989"—Contents p.
    Includes index
    ISBN 0-471-56066-9
        1. Cancer—Nutritional aspects—Congresses.   2. Cancer—
Prevention—Congresses.   3. Vitamins—Therapeutic use—Congresses.
I. Laidlaw, Stewart A.   II. Swendseid, Marian E.   III. Gladys Emerson
—UCLA Clinical Nutrition Research Unit Symposium (1989 : UCLA)
IV. Series.
RC268.45.V57   1991
616.99'405—dc20   90–44657
                                                                        CIP

Dedicated to the memory of

Gladys A. Emerson,

renowned nutrition scientist of the

vitamin discovery era

Contents

Contributors

Mary P. Carpenter, Ph.D., Department of Molecular Toxicology, Oklahoma Medical Research Foundation, and Department of Biochemistry and Molecular Biology, University of Oklahoma Health Sciences Center, Oklahoma City, OK 73104 **[61]**

John Ellis, Titus County Memorial Hospital, Mt. Pleasant, TX 75455 **[103]**

Karl Folkers, Institute for Biomedical Research, University of Texas at Austin, Austin, TX 78712 **[103]**

E. Robert Greenberg, M.D., Dartmouth Medical School and Norris Cotton Cancer Center, Hanover, NH 03756 **[1]**

Peter Greenwald, M.D., Dr.P.H., Division of Cancer Prevention and Control, National Cancer Institute, National Institutes of Health, Bethesda, MD 20892 **[111]**

Masahiro Kizaki, M.D., Department of Medicine, Division of Hematology-Oncology, University of California at Los Angeles, Los Angeles, CA 90024 **[91]**

H. Phillip Koeffler, M.D., Department of Medicine, Division of Hematology-Oncology, University of California at Los Angeles, Los Angeles, CA 90024 **[91]**

Carlos L. Krumdieck, M.D., Ph.D., Department of Nutrition Sciences, University of Alabama at Birmingham, Birmingham, AL 35294 **[39]**

Stewart A. Laidlaw, Ph.D., Division of Medical Oncology, UCLA Schools of Medicine and Public Health, Harbor-UCLA Medical Center, Torrance, CA 90509 **[xi]**

B. Mathew, M.D., Regional Cancer Centre, Trivandrum, India **[15]**

M. Krishnan Nair, M.D., Regional Cancer Centre, Trivandrum, India **[15]**

The numbers in brackets are the opening page numbers of the contributors' articles.

ix

Kimiyo Nara, Institute for Biomedical Research, University of Texas at Austin, Austin, TX 78712 **[103]**

Yoshio Nara, Institute for Biomedical Research, University of Texas at Austin, Austin, TX 78712 **[103]**

Lionel A. Poirier, Ph.D., Division of Comparative Toxicology, National Center for Toxicological Research, Jefferson, AR 72079 **[51]**

R. Sankaranarayanan, M.D., Regional Cancer Centre, Trivandrum, India **[15]**

Zongxuan Shen, Institute for Biomedical Research, University of Texas at Austin, Austin, TX 78712 **[103]**

Hans F. Stich, Ph.D., Environmental Carcinogenesis Unit, British Columbia Cancer Research Centre, Vancouver, British Columbia V5Z 1L3, Canada **[15]**

Marian E. Swendseid, Ph.D., Division of Nutrition Sciences, UCLA School of Public Health, Los Angeles, CA 90024 **[xi]**

Hiroo Tamagawa, Institute for Biomedical Research, University of Texas at Austin, Austin, TX 78712 **[103]**

Ajit K. Verma, Ph.D., Department of Human Oncology, University of Wisconsin Clinical Cancer Center, Madison WI 53792 **[25]**

Ovid Yang, Titus County Memorial Hospital, Mt. Pleasant, TX 75455 **[103]**

Chun-qu Ye, Institute for Biomedical Research, University of Texas at Austin, Austin, TX 78712 **[103]**

Preface

Gladys Emerson was most renowned for her work on the isolation of Vitamin E, although this work was only one highlight of a long and distinguished career in nutrition. She was a leading figure of that exciting era when the vitamins were discovered and characterized and their role in the prevention of deficiency diseases was established. Evidence is now accumulating that certain vitamins may also play roles in reducing the risk of many chronic diseases, including certain types of cancer. This volume is intended to present current knowledge regarding the role of vitamins in cancer prevention. The chapters are developed from presentations at the UCLA Clinical Nutrition Research Unit–Gladys Emerson Memorial Symposium held at UCLA on March 2–3, 1989. Their topics range over basic laboratory research on specific individual vitamins, data derived from clinical studies of vitamins as preventive agents, and preliminary studies of potential effects of vitamin deficiency in cancer patients. In addition, Chapter 9, "The Future of Nutrition Research in Cancer Prevention," explores a more general approach to research in nutrition that may have an impact on reducing the risk of cancer.

It is apparent that establishing the relationships between vitamins and cancer prevention or treatment on a firm basis is indeed a complex task. It is hoped that this volume will encourage further research and understanding of this intriguing and important problem.

Stewart A. Laidlaw, Ph.D.
Marian E. Swendseid, Ph.D.

Vitamins and Cancer Prevention, pages 1–14
© *1991 Wiley-Liss, Inc.*

| 1 | # An Approach to Studying the Possible Effects of Carotenoids in Skin Cancer Prevention
E. Robert Greenberg, M.D. |

INTRODUCTION

For the past eight years my colleagues and I have been engaged in a randomized, controlled trial of beta-carotene as a preventive agent for non-melanoma skin cancer [1]. Although the study was designed to answer one narrowly focused question, it may provide a useful vantage point from which to view the entire field of nutritional prevention of cancer. Our reasons for undertaking this trial and our experience in its conduct illustrate several issues common in studies of nutrition and cancer, particularly investigations that assess vitamins in cancer prevention. In this chapter I briefly discuss the types of study linking vitamins to cancer etiology, paying special attention to evidence that carotenoids may prevent cancer. I also discuss why human skin cancer is an attractive focus for studies of vitamins and cancer. Lastly, I

Dartmouth Medical School and Norris Cotton Cancer Center, Hanover, New Hampshire 03756 describe the Skin Cancer Prevention Study, which is testing the efficacy of beta-carotene in this condition.

STUDY TYPES

Interest in a relationship between vitamins and human cancer comes from two principal lines of investigation. One is nonexperimental (i.e., epidemiological) studies of the occurrence of human cancer as it relates to place of residence (for international–correlational studies) and to reported dietary intake or measured blood levels of vitamins (in case-control and cohort studies). The other is experimental studies of animal models of carcinogenesis. Both epidemiological and laboratory studies provide useful and often complementary data on the role of vitamins in cancer etiology. However, for the reasons discussed below, they generally do not constitute a sufficient basis for prescription of specific vitamins as cancer preventives for the general public.

Much of the evidence supporting a role of diet in human cancer comes from observations that the rate of occurrence of specific cancers varies widely from country to country [2]. For some neoplasms the incidence and mortality rates may vary by a factor of 10 or more. For example, stomach cancer mortality in men age 55–64 ranges from about 150 per 100,000 in Japan to about 15 per 100,000 in U.S. whites. Several other tumors show ranges of variation in their rates similar to that for stomach cancer [3]. Sometimes the variation in rates of cancer occurrence is due to known risk factors. Thus, differences between countries in lung cancer mortality rates appear to be almost entirely explicable by differences in the history of cigarette smoking among older adults in these populations. Often, however, the prevalence of known risk factors cannot account for international differences in cancer occurrence, leaving a large residual, which conceivably might be explained by dietary factors [4]. The total amount of cancer in the United States that might be explicable by diet is unknown, although an informed estimate is about 35% [2].

Many investigators used food disappearance data to correlate cancer rates with national or regional consumption of particular nutrients. These correlational studies led to a number of intriguing hypotheses. Perhaps the most notable are relationships between fat consumption and mortality rates for cancers of the breast and colorectum [4]. Results such as these are often useful for initial exploration of hypotheses and for focusing further studies. It is not always the case, however, that relationships found in aggregate apply to individuals, so further and more detailed studies are always needed. Moreover, nutrition–cancer correlations discovered at the international level may relate to other factors, such as levels of physical activity, which could underlie any observation and confuse the results of the analysis. The presence of these "confounding" variables is always a major concern in the interpretation of international correlations.

In case-control studies the characteristics of patients with cancer are compared to those of a group of controls, who usually are selected from the disease-free population. These types of studies provide stronger evidence than international correlations because: (1) the data associating diet and cancer pertain to individuals rather than groups, and (2) there is more information on possible confounding factors. Case-control studies of diet and cancer do have a number of difficulties, however, These largely center on inaccuracy of information on nutrient intake as assessed by dietary history. Random variation (imprecision) of nutrient measurements obtained by dietary recall tends to blur distinctions between cases and controls regarding dietary intake and thus may diminish or obscure a true diet–cancer relationship. Systematic error (bias) in recall of diet is an even more troubling concern, for it can both obscure a true relationship or produce a spurious relationship in the data. A hypothetical example of the way bias could distort study results is that sick cancer cases may underestimate their intake of certain unappetizing foods (for many people cabbage and brussel sprouts fall into this category). The effect of this bias would produce a spurious inverse relationship between consumption of these unappetizing foods and cancer risk. Another concern in case-control studies is confusion of cause and effect. This is a major issue in studies involving blood vitamin levels since one must consider whether the presence of cancer led to reduced vitamin levels rather than vice versa. Despite these limitations, well-performed case-control studies are generally viewed as providing stronger information than international correlations regarding possible vitamin–cancer relationships [5].

Cohort studies involve large groups of subjects whose nutrient status is initially characterized and who are then followed over many years to assess the occurrence of cancer. These studies have one major advantage over case-control studies in that the presence of cancer cannot bias assessment of diet or nutritional levels (at least not if one discounts the initial years of follow-up when the effects of undiscovered cancer may be present). However, confounding variables are still a crucial consideration when assessing results from cohort studies. For example, a lower rate of cancer in persons with high fruit intake could be due to an anticancer effect of vitamin C, but it could also be a result of other lifestyle features, such as not smoking, lean body habitus, fiber consumption, and so on. Thus, in nonexperimental studies such as cohort studies and case-control studies it is impossible to isolate completely the effects of one vitamin from the possible effects of other related dietary and nondietary factors.

There is a wealth of information from experimental laboratory studies that pertain to possible anticancer effects of various vitamins. These types of studies have done much to advance our understanding of the basic biology of neoplasia, and they provide valuable guidance for framing hypotheses regarding prevention of human cancer. Laboratory studies are discussed extensively elsewhere in this symposium, and their contributions to our knowledge are evident. It is important to point out, however, that laboratory studies have limited utility in guiding public policy about vitamins and cancer. The relevance of most animal models of carcinogenesis to human cancer prevention is uncertain. Also, the range of noncancer effects that may occur in humans due to nutritional supplementation cannot be extrapolated reliably from the results of animal studies. Thus, while laboratory studies of chemical carcinogens have been used (with considerable dispute) for setting policies about food additives, I doubt that they will greatly influence decisions regarding prescription of vitamins as possible cancer preventives. Clearcut results from randomized, controlled clinical trials will likely be required before advising the public to take substances, such as vitamins, to prevent cancer.

EVIDENCE THAT CAROTENOIDS ARE ANTICARCINOGENIC

Given this background, what is the evidence that the group of plant pigments known as carotenoids may prevent human cancer? Beta-carotene, a 40-carbon carotenoid, which is a precursor of vitamin A, was proposed approximately 10 years ago to have anticancer activity based both on epidemiological and laboratory evidence [6,7]. Since that time, evidence from human and animal studies has increased, much of it supporting the hypothesis. These data have been reviewed extensively in recent publications [8–10] and are summarized below.

The most consistent evidence linking beta-carotene to lower risk of human cancer comes from dietary case-control studies. The great majority of studies indicate that cancer patients report lower consumption of fruits and vegetables (including those rich in beta-carotene) than do controls. The evidence of protection relates to a number of epithelial cancers, with the strongest data indicating a lower risk of lung cancer in persons with high fruit and vegetable consumption. Many of these studies involve carefully devised and administered dietary questionnaires. However, it is not clear from the investigations whether beta-carotene, or some other factor associated with fruit and vegetable consumption accounts for the lower risk. A more complete review of the results of case-control studies may be found in other sources [7,9,10].

Results of early case-control studies led investigators to examine possible anticancer effects of beta-carotene using data from cohort studies designed for studying other issues. Two approaches have been followed. One involved analysis of detailed dietary histories obtained at study entry for groups of subjects followed over many years. Six studies of this type have been reported (Table I) and all show at least some evidence of lower cancer risk in

TABLE I. Follow-Up Studies of Dietary Carotenoids and Cancer

Reference	Study group	Carotenoid measurement	Cancer site	Number of cases	Finding in relation to carotenoids
11	265,000 Japanese adults	Green/yellow vegetables eaten daily or less often	Lung (deaths)	807	SMR[a] lower
			Prostate (deaths)	63	SMR lower
12	2107 Male employees of Chicago electrical firm	Carotene index (quartiles)	Lung	33	Trend of lower incidence, $p = 0.003$
			All others	175	No relationship, $p = 0.68$
13	13,785 Men, 2928 women in Norway and United States	Vitamin A index (quartiles)	Lung	153	Trend of lower incidence, $p = 0.04$
14	1271 Massachusetts men and women	Green/yellow vegetable score (quartiles)	All sites (deaths)	42	Trend of lower mortality, $p = 0.01$
15	1,000,000 U. S. men and women	Fruits and juices frequency (3 groups)	Lung (deaths)	2952	Lower SMR
16	10,473 Elderly California men and women	Beta-carotene frequency (tertiles)	Lung	55	No difference
			Colon	110	No difference
			Bladder	58	Lower incidence, $p < 0.05$ (for women)
			Prostate	92	No difference
			Breast	123	No difference

*Standardized mortality ratio.

persons with high carotenoid intake. Again, the strongest evidence relates to lung cancer although there have been positive findings for bladder cancer, colorectal cancer, breast cancer, and cancers of all sites combined (Table I). In many studies the numbers of cancers of specific sites was relatively small, so a true protective effect may have been overlooked because of low study power. No dietary cohort study has indicated an increased risk of any cancer associated with carotenoid intake, thus not confirming findings in some case-control studies that vitamin A was associated with a higher risk of prostatic cancer [17].

The second approach to cohort studies involved analysis of carotenoid levels in blood specimens collected at study entry from groups whose cancer incidence or mortality was determined over succeeding years. In these studies banked frozen sera were analyzed for persons who had developed cancer and for selected controls, that is, cohort members who did not get cancer. Results of six studies of this type have been published in seven articles (Table II). All but one study indicate an inverse relationship between beta-carotene blood levels and subsequent risk of cancer. The one clearly negative study [19] was based on spectrophotometric determination of total carotenoids, whereas the others employed high-performance liquid chromatography (HPLC) determination of beta-carotene. In one study [24], total carotenoids were measured in addition to beta-carotene. Again, the most consistent and strongest inverse relationship between carotenoids and cancer was found for lung cancer, particularly in males. There was weaker and less consistent evidence of protection for cancers of other sites including the colorectum, bladder, and stomach (Table II).

Some of the concerns raised earlier for case-control studies also pertain to the cohort study results, so it is not clear whether the lower cancer risk associated with blood carotenoid levels relates to carotenoids themselves or to other factors associated with carotenoid intake or absorption. For example, beta-carotene blood levels are consistently found to be lower among people who currently smoke cigarettes [25]. Thus, at least some of the negative relationship between beta-carotene and lung cancer risk could be due to residual confounding by cigarette smoking. Also people with high intake of beta-carotene (or high blood levels) likely have higher intake of other possibly protective substances found in fruits and vegetables. There are many potential anticarcinogens in these foods, and blood levels of beta-carotene may simply be an indirect indicator of their consumption.

Only a limited number of human experimental studies of beta-carotene and carcinogens have been reported. One of the more intriguing findings concerns a reduction in micronuclei in oral cells among betel nut chewers treated with beta-carotene in combination with retinol [26]. These studies are discussed in detail elsewhere in this symposium.

TABLE II. Follow-Up Studies of Blood Carotenoids and Cancer

Reference	Study group	Carotenoid measurement	Cancer by site	Number of cases	Finding in relation to carotenoid levels[a]
18	4,224 Men in Basel	Plasma beta-carotene (case-control difference)	Lung (deaths)	35	Lower in cases, $p < 0.05$
			Stomach (deaths)	19	Lower in cases, NS
			Colorectum (deaths)	14	No difference
			All others (deaths)	47	No difference
19	10,940 U. S. men and women hypertensives	Total serum carotenoids (case-control difference)	Lung	17	No difference
			Breast	14	No difference
			Prostate	11	No difference
			Leukemia/ lymphoma	11	Higher in cases, $p = 0.05$
			Gastrointestinal	11	No difference
			Other sites	40	No difference
20	8,006 Japanese men in Hawaii	Serum beta-carotene, quintiles	Lung	74	Lower risk, $p = 0.04$
			Stomach	70	Possible lower risk, NS
			Colon	81	Possible lower risk, NS
			Rectum	32	No difference
			Bladder	27	No difference
21, 22	25,802 Maryland men and women	Serum beta-carotene, quintiles	Lung	99	Lower risk, $p = 0.04$
			Colon	72	No difference
23	22,000 London men	Serum beta-carotene, quintiles	Lung	50	Lower risk, $p = 0.008$
			Colorectum	30	No significant difference for
			Stomach	13	any site but mean values for
			Bladder	15	cases lower than that for
			CNS	17	controls
			Skin	56	
			Other sites	90	
			All sites	271	Lower risk
24	12,866 American men at risk of heart disease	Serum total carotenoids and beta-carotene (quintiles)	Lung	66	Lower risk, $p = 0.03$ for total carotenoids, 0.08 for beta-carotene
			All sites	156	No significant difference

[a]NS = $p > 0.05$.

LABORATORY INVESTIGATIONS

Matthew-Roth [8] and Moon [27] reviewed experimental evidence for a protective effect of beta-carotene in several animal models of carcinogenesis. Efficacy has been found in a mouse skin model involving induction by ultraviolet light (administered either alone or in conjunction with chemical promoters) in rat mammary cancer induced by dithimethylbenzanthracine (DMBA), in rat liver induced by *N*-nitrosodiethylamine (DEN), and in hamster lung induced by DEN. The importance of these results is that they provide a firmer basis for believing that carotenoids, including beta-carotene, may have similar anticancer effects in humans. The actual relevance of these animal cancer models to human cancer occurrence and prevention, however, is not known.

Other laboratory studies have investigated a possible mechanism for an anticarcinogenic effect of beta-carotene. The available evidence supports two activities that may be relevant. One is the ability of beta-carotene (and some other carotenoids) to deactivate reactive molecular species such as singlet oxygen, peroxide-free radicals, and organic-free radicals [28]. The other important finding concerns possible immune enhancement resulting from beta-carotene administration [29]. Again, the importance of these types of studies is that they provide a firmer basis for hypothesizing that beneficial effects might occur in humans.

NONMELANOMA SKIN CANCER

Nonmelanoma skin cancers (NMSCs) affect approximately 500,000 people each year in the United States, making them the most common cancers occurring in our population [30]. Almost all NMSCs are either basal cell carcinomas (BCC) or squamous cell carcinomas (SCC). Of these, BCC is the most common occurring about 5–10 times more frequently than SCC. Skin cancers occur primarily on exposed areas of the skin with about 80% found on the face or head and about 5% on the upper extremities. Incidence rates are much higher in caucasians and among populations living at lower latitudes. Nonmelanoma skin cancers very rarely metastasize and they tend to cause disfigurement but not death. The most important known risk factors for NMSC are sunlight exposure and skin type (with highest risk found in persons who burn rather than tan when exposed to the sun). Ionizing radiation, certain chemical exposures, and chronic inflammation (due to injury or infection) are also risk factors, but probably account for a small minority of NMSC occurrence in the United States. The effect of diet or of nutritional factors has not been investigated to any extent.

Human NMSC is an excellent condition in which to test the possible preventive effects of carotenoids. Nonmelanoma skin cancer patients are relatively frequent and the risk of developing another skin cancer is high (approximately 10% per year) [31]. Nonmelanoma skin cancer can be readily detected by dermatological examination and biopsy. Also, high risk patients do not require intensive preventive efforts as do patients at risk of more lethal cancers. Lastly, the strongest laboratory evidence for an anticancer effect of beta-carotene and other carotenoids comes from studies of animal skin cancer [8]. For these reasons, it appeared that a clinical trial to test whether beta-carotene can prevent nonmelanoma skin cancer would be feasible and capable of providing important information on the possibility that carotenoids such as beta-carotene can prevent other human cancers.

THE SKIN CANCER PREVENTION STUDY

The hypothesis that beta-carotene would prevent cancer thus rested on a foundation of investigation from laboratory animals and human epidemiological studies. Although this information provided a strong basis for embarking on human investigations, it clearly was not adequate to support a recommendation that people take beta-carotene to prevent cancer [32]. This type of advice could best come from randomized, controlled trials. In 1982, our group therefore began a multicenter, randomized clinical trial testing whether oral ingestion of 50 mg of beta-carotene per day would reduce the time to occurrence of a first new NMSC in patients who recently had such a tumor removed. The study was undertaken with support from the U. S. National Cancer Institute and involved participating clinical centers at the University of California at Los Angeles, University of California Medical School at San Francisco, University of Minnesota Schools of Medicine and Public Health in Minneapolis, and the Dartmouth Medical School in Hanover, New Hampshire. The study was organized with a coordinating center in Dartmouth and clinical centers at all four institutions (Fig. 1). The clinical centers were responsible for recruiting patients, dispensing study agents, maintaining follow-up, performing dermatological examinations and biopsying suspicious skin lesions, drawing and shipping blood specimens, and reporting possible side effects. The coordinating center oversaw progress and funding. The coordinating center also performed laboratory analyses, dermatopathology slide review, study agent dispensation (obtaining, packaging, labeling, and mailing study capsules and calendar packs), data management, and statistical analyses (Fig. 1).

The study was directed by an executive committee composed of investigators at each of the clinical centers and the investigators at the coordinating center. Responsibility for reviewing unblinded data with regard to possible toxicity and efficacy was assigned to a Safety and Data Monitoring Committee composed of four outside consultants. This was the only group having access to unblinded data.

Beginning in February 1983, our group began to identify potentially eligible patients by reviewing reports of dermatopathology examinations in the clinical centers. A small number of patients learned of the study on their own

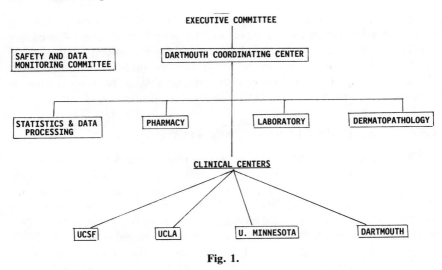

Fig. 1.

and asked to be entered. Patients were deemed eligible if they had at least one biopsy-proven NMSC since 1 January 1980, agreed not to take vitamin supplements containing vitamin A (or beta-carotene), were not vegan vegetarians, were under 85 years of age, and did not have any conditions that might limit their ability to participate in the study or that indicated an unusual type of NMSC (e.g., basal cell nevus syndrome, xeroderma pigmentosum, or arsenic exposure).

In 3 years of recruitment we identified 5232 potentially eligible subjects. Approximately one half of these were not interested in participating and about 15% could not be contacted to assess their interest. A total of 1968 patients entered into a placebo run-in phase to test their ability to adhere to study procedures. Of these 163 (8%) were not randomized because they lost interest in continuing in the study or because they appeared unlikely to follow the study regimen (usually because they took less than 80% of the prescribed placebo capsules). The remaining 1805 patients were assigned at random to take capsules containing either 50 mg of beta-carotene (BASF-Wyandotte, Michigan) (N = 913) or an identical-appearing placebo (N = 892). Capsules were mailed in calendar packs every 4 months with instructions to take one daily. Patients completed questionnaires three times per year regarding illnesses, possible treatment-associated symptoms, whether they took their capsules, their consumption of vegetables, use of vitamins, and any skin biopsies performed in the interval since the last questionnaire. They were scheduled to return for complete examination at the clinical centers by study dermatologists on an annual basis.

At the annual visits and at any interval visits study dermatologists removed all NMSC suspected lesions. These were prepared for pathology and examined locally, and then the pathology slides were reviewed by the coordinating center dermatopathologist. Major disagreements between assessments by the local and coordinating center pathologists were resolved by a third dermatopathologist. At the annual visits a blood sample was obtained for beta-carotene and retinol determination using HPLC [33,34].

Throughout the course of the study compliance with the treatment regimen was good. This was assessed both by questionnaire in which more than 80% of patients reported taking at least 50% of their capsules, and by measurement of blood levels of beta-carotene. The average plasma beta-carotene level of patients assigned to the active treatment group increased more than eightfold, from 176 to over 1600 ng/ml. The plasma beta-carotene level in the placebo group remained virtually unchanged. There was not a clinically significant increase in plasma retinol levels following beta-carotene administration for 1 year [1].

LESSONS FROM THE STUDY

In our initial experience with this trial we learned much that may be useful in the conduct of similar studies. A major discovery was that only a minority of patients who were eligible for the study chose to enroll. A principal reason given for not entering the study was an unwillingness to discontinue taking vitamin A preparations. Vitamin use is frequent among American adults, and many people are already convinced that taking vitamins will lower their risk of cancer, despite the lack of firm evidence that this is true. Other potential study subjects argued that vitamins were unlikely to be harmful, so why not take them on the chance there would be a benefit. Clearly there is a need to educate the public better about the known effects of vitamin intake.

A second lesson from the study was that careful selection of study subjects and continued instruction could result in high levels of cooperation. Persons who drop out of a study or do not comply with the prescribed treatment can seriously compromise the ability of an investigation to detect a true difference. We found the placebo run-in period to be helpful in that it allowed us to identify, before randomization, 163 people who almost certainly would not have complied with the study regimen had they been randomized. Study coordinators at each clinical center deserved much of the credit for continued cooperation of study subjects. These coordinators maintained close personal contact with patients and went to great lengths to ensure that study participants were well informed and made to feel important to the success of the study [35].

We also learned from this study that participation could be strongly affected by illnesses that occurred during the course of investigation but which were unrelated to either the study treatment or outcome. The population we studied included a high proportion of older people, many of whom already had one or more chronic, disabling conditions. When these conditions worsened, or when subjects acquired a new illness, participation in our study declined. One problem was that participants tended to blame study agents or stopping vitamins for any new symptom or illness occurring after randomization, no matter how remote the connection might be. In our data, reports of most types of symptoms were as frequent in the placebo group as in the actively treated group; nevertheless, patients ascribed these symptoms to their study participation and quickly considered stopping capsules and/or starting multivitamins. Many participants became so ill from a variety of conditions that they were unable to deal with the demands of participating in the trial. Preventing cancer became a low priority for people who were suffering under the burden of chronic illness.

CONCLUSIONS

Evidence from epidemiological studies and from animal studies strongly supports the notion that carotenoids may prevent cancer, but randomized controlled trials in humans are essential to resolve the issue of whether carotenoids should be prescribed for this purpose. Despite the difficulties encountered in conducting one such trial, the Skin Cancer Prevention Study, its progress was ultimately satisfactory. It achieved a clear contrast between the plasma beta-carotene levels of treated and untreated groups, and follow-up was excellent. For these reasons we think it has a high likelihood of providing a clear test of the hypothesis regarding an effect of beta-carotene on time to occurrence of first new nonmelanoma skin cancer. The results of this study and other clinical trials of beta-carotene in cancer should be published over the coming few years. At that time, there will be a much stronger basis for assessing the potential role of carotenoids in preventing human cancer.

REFERENCES

1. Greenberg ER, Baron JA, Stevens MM, Stukel TA, Mandel JS, Spencer SK, Elias PM, Lowe N, Nierenberg DW, Bayrd G, Vance JC, the Skin Cancer Prevention Study Group (1989): The Skin Cancer Prevention Study: design of a clinical trial of beta-carotene among persons at high risk for nonmelanoma skin cancer. Contr Clin Trials 10:153–166.
2. Doll R, Peto R (1981): "The Causes of Cancer: Quantitative Estimates of Avoidable Risks of Cancer in the United States Today." New York: Oxford University Press.

3. Kurihara M, Aoki K, Tominaga S (1984): "Cancer Mortality Statistics in the World." Nagoya, Japan: The University of Nagoya Press.

4. Armstrong B, Doll R (1975): Environmental factors and cancer incidence and mortality in different countries, with special reference to dietary practices. Int J Cancer 15:617–631.

5. Zaridze DG, Muir CS, McMichael AJ (1985): Diet and cancer: value of different types of epidemiological studies. Nutr Cancer 7:155–166.

6. Mathews-Roth MM (1980): Carotenoid pigments as antitumor agents. In Nelson JD, Grassi C (eds). "Current Chemotherapy and Infectious Disease." Washington, DC: The American Society for Microbiology, pp 1503–1505.

7. Peto R, Doll R, Buckley JD, Sporn MB (1981): Can dietary beta-carotene materially reduce human cancer rates? Nature 290:201–208.

8. Mathews-Roth MM (1989): Beta-carotene, canthaxanthin, and phytoene. In Moon TE, Micozzi MS (eds): "Nutrition and Cancer Prevention: Investigating the Role of Micronutrients." New York and Basel: Marcel Dekker, pp 273–290.

9. Ziegler RG (1989): A review of epidemiologic evidence that carotenoids reduce the risk of cancer. J Nutr 119:116–122.

10. Wald N (1987): Retinol, beta-carotene and cancer. Cancer Surveys 6:635–651.

11. Hirayama T (1979): Diet and cancer. Nutr Cancer 1:67–81.

12. Shekelle RB, Liu S, Raynor WJ, Jr, Lepper M, Maliza C, Rossof AH (1981): Dietary vitamin A and risk of cancer in the Western Electric Study. Lancet 2:1185–1189.

13. Kvale G, Bjelke E, Gart JJ (1983): Dietary habits and lung cancer risk. Int J Cancer 31:397–405.

14. Colditz GA, Branch LG, Lipnick RJ, Willett WC, Rosner B, Posner BM, Hennekens CH (1985): Increased green and yellow vegetable intake and lowered cancer deaths in an elderly population. Am J Clin Nutr 41:32–36.

15. Long-de W, Hammond EC (1985): Lung cancer, fruit, green salad and vitamin pills. Chinese Med J 98:206–210.

16. Paganini-Hill A, Chao A, Ross RK, Henderson BE (1987): Vitamin A, β-carotene, and the risk of cancer: a prospective study. J Natl Cancer Inst 443–448.

17. Kolonel LN, Hankin JH, Yoshizawa CN (1987): Vitamin A and prostatic cancer in elderly men: enhancement of risk. Cancer Res 47:2982–2985.

18. Stahelin HB, Rosel F, Buess E, Brubacher G (1984): Cancer, vitamins, and plasma lipids: prospective Basel study. J Natl Cancer Inst 73:1463–1468.

19. Willett WC, Polk BF, Underwood BA, Stampfer MJ, Pressel S, Rosner B, Taylor JA, Schneider K (1984): Relation of serum vitamins A and E and carotenoids to the risk of cancer. N Engl J Med 310:430–434.

20. Nomura AMY, Stemmermann GN, Heilbrun LK, Salkeld RM, Vuilleumier JP (1985): Serum vitamin levels and the risk of cancer of specific sites in men of Japanese ancestry in Hawaii. Cancer Res 45:2369–2372.

21. Menkes MS, Comstock GW, Vuilleumier JP, Helsing KJ, Rider AA, Brookmeyer R (1986): Serum beta-carotene, vitamins A and E, selenium, and the risk of lung cancer. N Engl J Med 315:1250–1254.

22. Schober SE, Comstock GW, Helsing KJ, Salkeld RM, Morris JS, Rider AA, Brookmeyer R (1987): Serologic precursors of cancer. I. Prediagnostic serum nutrients and colon cancer risk. Am J Epidemiol 126:1033–1041.

23. Wald NJ, Thompson SG, Densem JW, Boreham J, Bailey A (1988): Serum Beta-carotene and subsequent risk of cancer: Results from the BUPA study. Br J Cancer 57:428–433.

24. Connett JE, Kuller LH, Kjelsberg MO, Polk BF, Collins G, Rider A, Hulley SB (1989): Relationship between carotenoids and cancer. Cancer 64:126–134.

25. Nierenberg DW, Stukel TA, Baron JA, Dain BJ, Greenberg ER (1989): Determinants of plasma levels of beta-carotene and retinol. Am J Epidemiol 130:511–521.

26. Stich HF, Rosin MP (1984): Reduction with vitamin A and beta-carotene administration of proportion of micronucleated buccal mucosa cells in Asian betel nut and tobacco chewers. Lancet 1:1204–1206.

27. Moon RC (1989): Comparative aspects of carotenoids and retinoids as chemopreventive agents for cancer. J Nutr 119:127–134.

28. Krinsky NI (1989): Carotenoids as chemopreventive agents. Prev Med 18:592–602.

29. Bendich A, Shapiro SS (1986): Effect of beta-carotene and canthaxanthin on the immune response of the rat. J Nutr 116:2254–2262.

30. Scotto J, Fraumeni JF, Jr (1982): Skin (Other than Melanoma). In Schottenfeld D, Fraumeni JF, Jr (eds). ''Cancer and Epidemiology and Prevention.'' Philadelphia: Saunders, pp 966–1011.

31. Robinson JK (1987): Risk of developing another basal cell carcinoma. Cancer 60:118–120.

32. Hennekens CH (1986): Micronutrients and cancer prevention. N Engl J Med 315:1288–1289.

33. Nierenberg DW (1984): ''Determination of serum and plasma concentrations of retinol using high-performance liquid chromatography. J Chromatogr 311:239–248.

34. Nierenberg DW (1985): Serum and plasma beta-carotene levels measured with an improved method of high-performance liquid chromatography. J Chromatogr 339:273–278.

35. Stevens M, Greenberg ER, Baron JA (1989): Practical Aspects of Cancer Prevention Trials. In Micozzi MS, Moon TE (eds). ''Nutrition and Cancer Prevention: The Role of Micronutrients.'' New York: Marcel Dekker, pp 513–532.

Vitamins and Cancer Prevention, pages 15–24
© 1991 Wiley-Liss, Inc.

2 | Vitamin A and Beta-Carotene: Long-Term Protective Effects in Oral Leukoplakia

Hans F. Stich, Ph.D.
B. Mathew, M.D.
R. Sankaranarayanan, M.D.
M. Krishnan Nair, M.D.

INTRODUCTION

The administration of chemopreventive agents as a means of reducing cancer is currently attracting considerable attention. Clinical trials have been conducted using beta-carotene [1–5]; or a retinoid (e.g., 3,6–10] to protect against the development of precancerous lesions and against the progression towards malignant cancers. Large scale prevention studies are costly, require a multidisciplinary approach, are time consuming, and are difficult to control, considering the differences in dietary habits and lifestyle patterns within a participating study cohort [6]. Despite considerable efforts in several coun-

Environmental Carcinogenesis Unit, British Columbia Cancer Research Centre, Vancouver, British Columbia V52 1L3, Canada (H.F.S.); and Regional Cancer Centre, Trivandrum, India (B.M., R.S., M.K.N.)

tries, the outcome of intervention trials on precancerous lesions of various tissues, including colon, oral cavity, cervix, lung, esophagus, and skin, still remains unknown [11,12]. To improve on this situation, the use of various precancerous cell markers as intermediate endpoints has been suggested. Micronuclei have been found to be suitable as internal dosimeters for revealing genotoxic damage in human tissues exposed to carcinogens [13–18], and for following the response of individuals to chemopreventive agents [2,18–22]. The term "micronuclei" has been applied to a variety of Feulgen-positive structures, which are located in the cytoplasm and have no connection to the main cell nucleus. They result from acentric chromosomes, chromatid fragments, or aberrant chromosomes that have not been included in the main nucleus, and thus appear as separate entitites in the cytoplasm. The use of micronucleus occurrence frequencies as an intermediate endpoint has the following advantages. The micronucleus test can be performed on several hundred exfoliated cells or on tissue sections, thus permitting a comparison with histological changes, and it can be submitted to an automated scoring system [23,24]. In this study, we made use of this phenomenon as a marker to estimate the maintenance of an induced protective effect after withdrawal of the vitamin regime. The protective effect was induced by administration of either beta-carotene or a mixture of beta-carotene and vitamin A in heavy doses. As in our previous studies, we used tobacco–areca nut chewers as subjects [2,19,21].

CANCER-CAUSING HABITS OF TRIAL PARTICIPANTS

For the intervention studies, tobacco–areca nut-chewing fishermen near Trivandrum (Kerala, India) were selected because of their homogeneous characteristic lifestyle patterns. The composition of the chewing mixtures was simple and relatively uniform, consisting of tobacco, a piece of areca nut (*Areca catechu* L.), betel leaf (*Piper betle* L.), and slaked lime. Compounds that could conceivably be involved in carcinogenesis of the oral mucosa of the chewers are tobacco-specific nitrosamines, including N'nitrosonornicotine (NNN) and N-nitrosoanatabine (NAT) [25], areca nut-specific nitrosamines, including N-nitrosoguvacoline (NGCO), N-nitrosoguvacine (NG), and 3-(methylnitrosamino)propionitrile (MNPN) [26,27], areca nut-derived polyphenolics, such as delphinidin, catechin, cyanadin, and tannic acids [28], aqueous areca nut extracts [29,30], and arecoline, which are promoters rather than initiators [31]. Due to the alkaline saliva resulting from the use of slaked lime in the betel quid, the phenolics from the areca nut will generate free radicals that may directly affect the oral mucosal cells. Elevated H_2O_2 levels can actually be found in the saliva of betel quid chewers [29]. We have estimated that the amount of NNN plus NAT would reach approximately 66.5 μg/day, and the amount of NG would be 2.3 μg/day in the saliva of betel quid chewers [32]. Furthermore, tobacco-specific nitrosamines derived from bidi (local cigarettes) smoking and a considerable intake of alcoholic beverages contribute to the load of carcinogens, cancer promoters, or cocarcinogens affecting the oral mucosa of the trial participants.

ORAL MUCOSAL CELLS WITH MICRONUCLEI AS AN ENDPOINT

In this study, micronuclei were used as an intermediate endpoint. Micronuclei result from chromatid or chromosome fragments caused by aberrations that occur in the dividing cell population of the basal cell layer of the oral mucosa. Micronucleated cells were found to be increased in the oral mucosa of individuals engaged in cancer-causing habits such as the chewing of various tobacco-containing mixtures [18,24,31] or snuff dipping [20]. These chromatid aberrations, which occur continuously over the many years of tobacco chewing or snuff dipping lead to the continuous formation of cells with a reshuffled genome, including deletions and translocations of gene sequences. It is likely, although unproven, that these events may result in the loss of genes, gene amplification, or in changes of genetic expression, which appear to be phenomena involved in neoplastic transformation. Since the formation of micronuclei may indicate an event in the chain of processes leading to the development of a neoplastic phenotype, they may be acceptable markers to reveal the response of a tissue to the action of chemopreventive agents.

REDUCTION OF PRENEOPLASTIC ORAL LESIONS FOLLOWING ADMINISTRATION OF BETA-CAROTENE OR BETA-CAROTENE PLUS VITAMIN A

The twice weekly administration of beta-carotene (180 mg/week) or beta-carotene (180 mg/week) plus vitamin A (100,000 IU/week) to tobacco–areca nut chewers reduced the frequency of exfoliated buccal mucosal cells with micronuclei [21], induced the remission of oral leukoplakia in a certain percentage of treated individuals [2], and prevented the formation of new leukoplakias within the 6-month trial period (Table I).

MAINTENANCE OF THE PROTECTIVE EFFECT

Following withdrawal of the chemopreventive treatment, the frequency of micronucleated cells started to increase in the oral mucosa, reaching, within

ILE I. Response of Oral Leukoplakias and Micronucleated Oral Mucosal Cells of acco–Areca Nut Chewers to the Administration of Chemopreventive Agents for 6 Months

Treatment	Individuals (n)	Individuals with		Individuals (n)	Cells with micronuclei	
		Remission	New leukoplakia		Before treatment	After treatment
Placebo	33	1 (3.0%)	7 (21.2%)	30	3.80 ± 0.23	4.00 ± 0.24
Beta-carotene (180 mg/week)	27	4 (14.8%)	4 (14.8%)	26	4.35 ± 0.27	0.86 ± 0.08
Vitamin A (100,000 IU/week) + beta-carotene (180 mg/week)	51	14 (27.5%)	4 (7.8%)	40	4.18 ± 0.22	1.00 ± 0.11

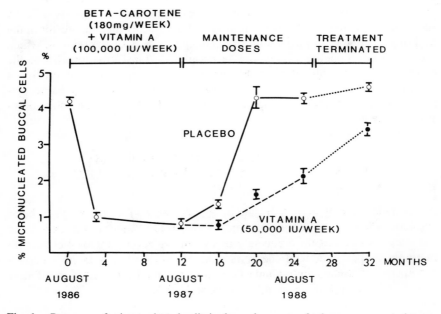

Fig. 1. Response of micronucleated cells in the oral mucosa of tobacco–areca nut chewers (61 individuals) to a 12-month administration of beta-carotene plus vitamin A, followed by 13 months of a maintenance dose of vitamin A and an additional 7 months without any treatment. After the first 12 months, the 61 treated individuals were split into a group receiving placebo and a group receiving vitamin A (50,000 IU/week).

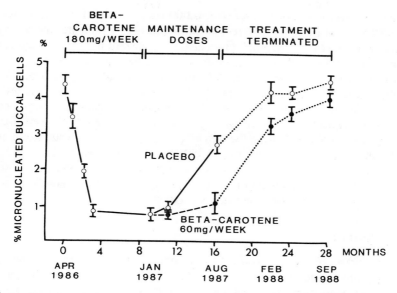

Fig. 2. Response of micronucleated cells in the oral mucosa of tobacco–areca nut chewers (60 individuals) to a 9-month administration of beta-carotene (180 mg/week), followed by 7 months of a maintenance dose of beta-carotene, and an additional 12 months without any treatment. After the first 9 months, the 60 treated individuals were split into a group receiving placebo and a group receiving beta-carotene (60 mg/week).

approximately 8 months, levels found in chewers before the onset of beta-carotene or beta-carotene plus vitamin A administration (Figs. 1 and 2). In this connection, it is important to note that all the trial participants continued to chew unabated throughout the trial and post-trial period. They chewed an average of approximately 11 times per day for 13 min per chew. Thus their oral mucosa remained continuously exposed to the mixture of cancer initiators and promoters. The return of chromatid or chromosome aberrations in the dividing basal cell layers that lead to the formation of micronuclei detectable in the sampled exfoliated oral mucosal cells after termination of the chemopreventive treatment is therefore not surprising.

We sought to examine whether the protective effect obtained with high carotenoid–vitamin A doses could be maintained over a prolonged period of time by the administration of lower doses of beta-carotene or nontoxic doses of vitamin A. Two experiments were carried out to address this. The frequency of micronucleated oral mucosal cells of chewers was reduced by a 12-month administration of beta-carotene (180 mg/week) plus vitamin A (100,000 IU/week). Thereafter, one group of tobacco–areca nut chewers was placed on lower doses of vitamin A (50,000 IU/week) for 13 months, and a second group on placebo. The results shown in Fig. 1 indicate that the low maintenance doses of vitamin A prevented the return of micronucleated cells to levels found in chewers prior to the onset of the intervention trial for at least 13 months. After the vitamin A treatment was terminated, the frequency of micronucleated cells increased again, approaching pretreatment levels after 7 additional months. The second experiment consisted of giving beta-carotene (180 mg/week) twice weekly to tobacco–areca nut chewers for 9 months, and then subdividing the treated group into a placebo subgroup and a subgroup receiving only 60 mg of beta-carotene per week (Fig. 2). All types of treatment were withdrawn after 7 months on the maintenance doses. In this study, the administration of vitamin A proved to be more effective than that of beta-carotene at the doses used.

DISCUSSION

Considerable evidence from clinical trials and experiments on animal models point to the chemopreventive effect of retinoids and beta-carotene [11,12,33]. However, the maintenance of this protective effect over a prolonged period of time after withdrawal of the treatment remains an unresolved issue. The main difficulty arises from the necessity of administering relatively high doses of a chemoprotective agent to obtain the remission of leukoplakias and a reduction in the frequency of micronucleated cells; the ensuing adverse effects that these therapeutic doses of retinoids can produce restrict the long-term use of the retinoids currently available [7,34]. Even the administration of larger doses of the nontoxic beta-carotene [35–37] may not be readily acceptable due to the undesirable coloration of the skin. Simple, economical methods to maintain a desirable effect over a prolonged timespan after the actual treatment period must be found. Our results on tobacco–areca nut chewers revealed the feasibility of extending a protective effect of beta-carotene and vitamin A by using doses that are considerably lower than those required to reduce the frequency of micronucleated buccal mucosal cells. Such low doses of vitamin A and/or beta-carotene, which did not lead to any detectable undesirable side-effects, were readily accepted by the trial participants. The method of choice appears to be the administration of relatively heavy chemopreventive doses for a short time to obtain a protective effect, followed by the maintenance of this protective effect with lower doses of vitamin A, and the return to a high-dose regime when the first signs of recurrence of the preneoplastic lesions become evident.

The alternation of heavy and low doses of vitamin A described above appears to be a suitable manner in which to prevent toxic side effects. Similarly, high doses of beta-carotene alternated with lower maintenance doses may avoid any undesirable coloration of the skin following supplementation [38,39]. Even if the toxicity and side effects of these agents can be eliminated using particular treatment regimes, numerous issues must be resolved before chemopreventive measures can be applied to larger population groups. The short- and long-term oral administration of capsules containing beta-carotene has revealed considerable interindividual variations in its increased plasma levels [40–43] and uptake by cells of the oral mucosa [44,45] or urogenital tract [46]. Weakly responding individuals may not attain sufficiently high doses of a chemopreventive agent that would convey a protective effect in the target tissue exposed to chemical carcinogens. Information on the percentage of individuals either not responding or responding weakly to a preventive agent would help in the interpretation of trial results. The identification of weak and strong responders could conceivably be used in the selection of population groups that are amenable to a chemopreventive approach. Furthermore, several factors, including cigarette smoking [47], alcohol consumption [44], and sex [48], can influence beta-carotene levels in plasma or tissue. Even if these results should prove to be due to different daily intakes of food products containing beta-carotene, they should be taken into account when the degree of response of a heterogeneous population group to a chemopreventive trial is estimated. Another unresolved issue is the restricted number of chemicals that have been tested for their chemopreventive potential. For example, of the large number of carotenoids in edible fruits and vegetables, only beta-carotene has been treated in human population groups. Other carotenoids, such as lycopene or zeaxanthin, which are ingested at levels comparable to those of beta-carotene, should be examined for their electron scavenging activity and their chemopreventive effect in model systems and in humans. Finally, the cumbersome, unreliable, and expensive administration of pills or capsules to large numbers of individuals at elevated risk for cancer, such as chewers of tobacco or tobacco-containing mixtures, should be replaced by equally effective but more economic methods. The potential for obtaining a relatively high intake of beta-carotene through the increased consumption of red palm oil [49], yellow varieties of sweet potatoes [50], and other vegetables rich in carotenoids has not been fully explored. In addition, simple food fortification with carotenoids and vitamin A must be introduced before a chemopreventive approach can be applied to large population groups engaged in cancer-causing habits.

ACKNOWLEDGMENTS

These studies were supported by the National Cancer Institute of Canada and by Hoffman-La Roche & Co., Basel, Switzerland. Dr. H.F. Stich is a

Terry Fox Cancer Research Scientist of the National Cancer Institute of Canada.

REFERENCES

1. Santamaria L, Benazzo L, Benazzo M, Bianchi A (1988): First clinical case-report (1980–1988) of cancer chemoprevention with beta-carotene plus canthaxanthin supplemented to patients after radical treatment. Med Biol Environ 16:945–950.
2. Stich HF, Rosin MP, Hornby AP, Mathew B, Sankaranarayanan R, Krishnan Nair M (1988): Remission of oral leukoplakias and micronuclei in tobacco/betel quid chewers treated with beta-carotene and with beta-carotene plus vitamin A. Int J Cancer 42:195–199.
3. Stich HF, Brunnemann KD, Mathew B, Sankaranarayanan R, Krishnan Nair M (1989): Chemopreventive trials with vitamin A and β-carotene: some unresolved issues. Prev Med 18:732–739.
4. Buring JE, Hennekens CH (1989): The possible role of beta-carotene in cancer prevention. Cancer Prev July:1–9.
5. Ziegler RG (1989): A review of epidemiologic evidence that carotenoids reduce the risk of cancer. J Nutr 119:116–122.
6. Hennekens CH, Mayrent SL, Willett W (1986): Vitamin A, carotenoids, and retinoids. Cancer 58:1837–1841.
7. Hong WK, Endicott J, Itri LM, Doos W, Batsakis JG, Bell R, Fofonoff S, Byers R, Atkinson EN, Vaughan C, Toth BB, Kramer A, Dimery IW, Skipper P, Strong S (1986): 13-cis-Retinoic acid in the treatment of oral leukoplakia. New Engl J Med 315:1501–1505.
8. Lippman SM, Kessler JF, Meyskens FL, Jr (1987): Retinoids as preventive and therapeutic anticancer agents (Part I). Cancer Treat Rep 71:391–405.
9. Lippman SM, Kessler JF, Meyskens FL (1987): Retinoids as preventive and therapeutic anticancer agents (Part II). Cancer Treat Rep 71:493–515.
10. Kraemer KH, DiGiovanna JJ, Moshell AN, Tarone RE, Peck GL (1988): Prevention of skin cancer in xeroderma pigmentosum with the use of oral isotretinoin. N Engl J Med 318:1633–1637.
11. Bertram JS, Kolonel LN, Meyskens FL, Jr (1987): Rationale and strategies for chemoprevention of cancer in humans. Cancer Res 47:3012–3031.
12. Temple NJ, Basu TK (1988): Does beta-carotene prevent cancer? A critical appraisal. Nutr Res 8:685–701.
13. Stich HF, Curtis JR, Parida BB (1982): Application of the micronucleus test to exfoliated cells of high cancer risk groups: tobacco chewers. Int J Cancer 30:553–559.
14. Stich HF, Stich W, Parida BB (1982): Elevated frequency of micronucleated cells in the buccal mucosa of individuals at high risk for oral cancer: betel quid chewers. Cancer Lett 17:125–134.
15. Stich HF, Rosin MP (1983): Micronuclei in exfoliated human cells as an internal dosimeter for exposures to carcinogens. In Stich HF (ed): "Carcinogens and Mutagens in the Environment," Vol II, "Naturally Occurring Compounds: Endogenous Formation and Modulation." Boca Raton, FL: CRC, pp 17–25.
16. Stich HF, Rosin MP (1985): Towards a more comprehensive evaluation of a genotoxic hazard in man. Mutation Res 150:43–50.
17. Fontham E, Correa P, Rodriguez E, Lin Y (1986): Validation of smoking history with the micronuclei test. In Hoffman D, Harris C (eds): "Mechanisms in Tobacco Carcinogene-

sis.'' Banbury Report 23. Cold Spring Harbor, NY: Cold Spring Harbor Laboratory, pp 113–119.

18. Stich HF (1987): Micronucleated exfoliated cells as indicators for genotoxic damage and as markers in chemoprevention trials. J Nutr Growth Cancer 4:9–18.

19. Stich HF, Stich W, Rosin MP, Vallejera MO (1984): Use of the micronucleus test to monitor the effect of vitamin A, beta-carotene and canthaxanthin on the buccal mucosa of betel nut/tobacco chewers. Int J Cancer 34:745–750.

20. Stich HF, Hornby AP, Dunn BP (1985): A pilot beta-carotene intervention trial with Inuits using smokeless tobacco. Int J Cancer 36:321–327.

21. Stich HF, Hornby AP, Mathew B, Sankaranarayanan R, Krishnan Nair M (1988): Response of oral leukoplakias to the administration of vitamin A. Cancer Lett 40:93–101.

22. Munoz N, Hayashi M, Lu JB, Wahrendorf J, Crespi M, Bosch FX (1987): Effect of riboflavin, retinol, and zinc on micronuclei of buccal mucosa and of esophagus: a randomized double-blind intervention study in China. J Natl Cancer Inst 79:687–691.

23. Callisen HH, Pincu M, Norman A (1986): Feasibility of automating the micronucleus assay. Anal Quant Cytol Histol 8:219–223.

24. Stich HF, Acton AB, Palcic B (1990): Towards an automated micronucleus assay as an internal dosimeter for carcinogen-exposed human population groups. In Band P (ed): ''Occupational Cancer Epidemiology.'' Recent Results in Cancer Research, Vol 120, Berlin, Heidelberg, New York: Springer-Verlag, pp 94–105.

25. Hoffmann D, Hecht SS (1985): Nicotine-derived *N*-nitrosamines and tobacco-related cancer: current status and future directions. Cancer Res 45:935–944.

26. Wenke G, Brunnemann KD, Hoffmann D, Bhide SV (1984): A study of betel quid carcinogenesis. IV. Analysis of the saliva of betel chewers: a preliminary report. J Cancer Res Clin Oncol 108:110–113.

27. Nair J, Ohshima H, Friesen M, Croisy A, Bhide SV, Bartsch H (1985): Tobacco-specific and betel nut-specific *N*-nitroso compounds: occurrence in saliva and urine of betel quid chewers and formation in vitro by nitrosation of betel quid. Carcinogenesis 6:295–303.

28. Stich HF, Bohm BA, Chatterjee K, Sailo JL (1983): The role of saliva-borne mutagens and carcinogens in the etiology of oral and esophageal carcinomas of betel nut and tobacco chewers. In Stich HF (ed): ''Carcinogens and Mutagens in the Environment,'' Vol III, ''Naturally Occurring Compounds: Epidemiology and Distribution.'' Boca Raton, FL: CRC, pp 43–58.

29. Stich HF, Anders F (1989): The involvement of reactive oxygen species in oral cancers of betel quid/tobacco chewers. Mutation Res 214:47–61.

30. Stich HF, Tsang SS (1989): Promoting activity of betel quid ingredients and their inhibition by retinol. Cancer Lett 45:71–77.

31. Stich HF, Tsang SS, Palcic B, Mathew B, Sankaranarayanan R, Krishnan Nair M (1990): The usefulness of in vitro assays and animal experiments in the design of chemopreventive protocols with beta-carotene and vitamin A on tobacco chewers. In Prasad KN (ed): ''Nutrients and Cancer Prevention.'' Clifton, NJ: Humana Press, pp 119–134.

32. Brunnemann KD, Hornby AP, Stich HF (1987): Tobacco-specific nitrosamines in the saliva of Inuit snuff dippers in the Northwest Territories of Canada. Cancer Lett 37:7–16.

33. Peto R, Doll R, Buckley JD, Sporn MB (1981): Can dietary beta-carotene materially reduce human cancer rates? Nature (London) 290:201–208.

34. Teelmann K (1989): Retinoids: toxicology and teratogenicity to date. Pharmacol Ther 40:29–43.

35. Heywood R, Palmer AK, Gregson RL, Hummler H (1985): The toxicity of beta-carotene. Toxicology 36:91–100.

36. Bendich A (1988): The safety of β-carotene. Nutr Cancer 11:207–214.
37. Mathews-Roth MM (1988): Lack of genotoxicity with beta-carotene. Toxicol Lett 41: 185–191.
38. Willett WC, Stampfer MJ, Underwood BA, Taylor JO, Hennekens CH (1983): Vitamins A, E, and carotene: effects of supplementation on their plasma levels. Am J Clin Nutr 38:559–566.
39. Micozzi MS, Brown ED, Taylor PR, Wolfe E (1988): Carotenodermia in men with elevated carotenoid intake from foods and β-carotene supplements. Am J Clin Nutr 48: 1061–1064.
40. Meyer JC, Grundmann HP, Seeger B, Schnyder UW (1985): Plasma concentrations of beta-carotene and canthaxanthin during and after stopping intake of a combined preparation. Dermatologica 171:76–81.
41. Dimitrov NV, Boone CW, Hay MB, Whetter P, Pins M, Kelloff GJ, Malone W (1986): Plasma beta-carotene levels—kinetic patterns during administration of various doses of beta-carotene. J Nutr Growth Cancer 3:227–237.
42. Dimitrov NV, Meyer C, Ullrey DE, Chenoweth W, Michelakis A, Malone W, Boone C, Fink G (1988): Bioavailability of β-carotene in humans. Am J Clin Nutr 48:298–304.
43. Costantino JP, Kuller LH, Begg L, Redmond CK, Bates MW (1988): Serum level changes after administration of a pharmacologic dose of β-carotene. Am J Clin Nutr 48:1277–1283.
44. Stich HF, Hornby AP, Dunn BP (1986): Beta-carotene levels in exfoliated mucosa cells of population groups at low and elevated risk for oral cancer. Int J Cancer 37:389–393.
45. Gilbert AM, Stich HF, Rosin MP, Davison AJ (1990): Variations in the uptake of beta-carotene in the oral mucosa of individuals after 3 days of supplementation. Int J Cancer 45:855–859.
46. Cameron LM, Rosin MP, Stich HF (1989): Use of exfoliated cells to study tissue-specific levels of beta-carotene in humans. Cancer Lett 45:203–207.
47. Chow CK, Thacker RR, Changchit C, Bridges RB, Rehm SR, Humble J, Turbek J (1986): Lower levels of vitamin C and carotenes in plasma of cigarette smokers. J Am Coll Nutr 5:305–312.
48. Ito Y, Sasaki R, Minohara M, Otani M, Aoki K (1987): Quantitation of serum carotenoid concentrations in healthy inhabitants by high-performance liquid chromatography. Clin Chim Acta 169:197–208.
49. Goh SH, Choo YM, Ong SH (1985): Minor constituents of palm oil. J Am Oil Chem Soc 62:237–240.
50. Wang H (1982): The breeding of sweet potatoes for human consumption. In Villareal RL, Griggs TD (eds): "Sweet Potato: Proceedings of the First International Symposium." Shanhua, Tainan, Taiwan: Asian Vegetable Research and Development Center, pp 297–311.

Vitamins and Cancer Prevention, pages 25–37
© *1991 Wiley-Liss, Inc.*

3	# Modulation of Carcinogenesis by Vitamin A and Its Analogs (Retinoids)

Ajit K. Verma, Ph.D.

INTRODUCTION

Vitamin A, a fat-soluble vitamin, plays an essential role in the visual cycle and is required in normal growth of bone, reproduction, embryonic development and differentiation of epithelial tissue [1–5]. Retinol is a circulating form of vitamin A and is generated from either dietary β-carotene or retinyl esters. In the target tissue, retinol is metabolized to the aldehyde retinal, which is further oxidized irreversibly to retinoic acid [3]. Retinoic acid is necessary to maintain the normal pathway of growth and differentiation of epithelial tissues but it cannot replace retinal to support visual and reproduc-

Department of Human Oncology, University of Wisconsin Clinical Cancer Center, Madison, Wisconsin 53792

tion functions [1]. It is noteworthy that vitamin A deficiency in hamsters results in the keratinization of tracheobronchial epithelium (squamous metaplasia). In this preneoplastic condition, normal columnar ciliated and mucus cells are replaced by squamous cells which produce specific keratin. Squamous metaplasia can be reversed by vitamin A supplementation [6]. Since neoplastic transformation usually results in the loss of normal cellular differentiation and retinoic acid is an essential micronutrient that controls cellular differentiation, it is evident that retinoic acid and its analogs (retinoids) may be promising agents for prevention and treatment of human cancer. Evidence is presented in this chapter that retinoids are highly selective chemopreventive agents and the mechanisms underlying their target organ specificity may involve specific nuclear receptor-mediated gene expression.

VITAMIN A DEFICIENCY AND SUSCEPTIBILITY TO CARCINOGENESIS

Epidemiological studies provide evidence of an association between vitamin A consumption and risk of some human cancers [7]. A few examples will be cited. In a case-controlled study, 364 primary lung cancer patients and 627 population controls, matched by age and sex, were interviewed for dietary intake of vitamin A, carotene, and vitamin C. Dietary vitamin A and carotene intake were found to be inversely correlated with lung cancer risk in males but not in females of the multiethnic population of Hawaii [8]. Mettlin et al. [9] interviewed 292 white male patients with lung cancer and 801 control patients with nonrespiratory, nonneoplastic diseases for diet and smoking history. Analysis of data from epidemiologic questionnaires indicate an association between vitamin A intake and lower risk of lung cancer in heavy smokers. Of special interest is the observation that low vitamin A intake is associated not only with an increased risk of lung cancer but also with malignancies at other sites. In a multisite case-control study by Middleton et al. [7], groups of males and females were evaluated for dietary vitamin A and cancer risk at 25 sites. Dietary vitamin A was associated with lower risk for cancers of the mouth, pharynx, larynx, esophagus, and lung among males and for bladder cancer among females. A number of recent reports, including a multiple risk factor intervention trial, have substantiated the fact that there is an inverse relationship between dietary intake of carotenoids and cancer [8,10]. The results of epidemiologic studies are interesting but should be interpreted with caution because of the fact that diet is a complex mixture of many nutrients and a nutrient other than vitamin A or the combination of vitamin A with other diet components may be associated with the results obtained. However, data from experimental animals also support the concept that vitamin A deficiency increases susceptibility to the induction of cancer of lung, bladder, and colon in animals [11,12].

RETINOIDS AS MODULATORS OF CARCINOGENESIS
Retinoids Are Antitumor Promoters

Data from experimental animals indicate that carcinogenesis involves qualitatively different steps: initiation, promotion, and progression [13]. These steps in carcinogenesis have been extensively studied in the mouse skin system [14]. Mouse skin tumor initiation can be accomplished by a single application of a carcinogen at a dose sufficiently small that it will not lead to the induction of visible tumors during the life span of the animal. Many tumors, however, develop following repeated and prolonged applications to the initiated skin of another chemical known as a tumor promoter. Application of a tumor promoter alone rarely elicits tumors; it is only following initiation that promoters elicit tumors. 12-O-Tetradecanoylphorbol-13-acetate (TPA), a component of croton oil, is a potent mouse skin tumor promoter. The multiple steps in carcinogenesis have also been demonstrated in organs other than skin including liver, urinary bladder, colon, and breast [14,15].

Retinoic acid and certain of its analogs have been shown to inhibit the induction of cancer in urinary bladder, breast, and skin [16–19]. Evidence indicates that retinoids inhibit carcinogenesis by interference with the promotion and not with the initiation stage of carcinogenesis [17]. The effects of retinoids on the stages of carcinogenesis have been investigated in detail in the mouse skin system [20]. Retinoic acid did not affect the initiation, but inhibited the promotion of mouse skin tumor formation. In this study, groups of female CD-1 mice were treated with 68 nmol of retinoic acid 1 hr prior to, concurrent with, or several days after initiation with 7,12-dimethyl-benz[*a*]anthracene (DMBA); 2 weeks after initiation, the mice were promoted with 17 nmol of TPA twice weekly. These treatments resulted in an insignificant effect on both the number of papillomas per mouse and the number of mice bearing papillomas. In contrast, a single application of 68 nmol of retinoic acid 1 hr before each promotion treatment with TPA resulted in a 60% reduction in the tumor multiplicity, while 47% of the mice did not bear papillomas. A similar degree of inhibition of mouse skin tumor promotion by retinoic acid was observed using female SENCAR mice and benzo[*a*]pyrene as an initiator. Retinoic acid also inhibited the incidence of mouse skin carcinomas [21].

For inhibition of skin tumor formation, retinoic acid treatments have to be scheduled close to TPA applications. A specific example is the observation that retinoic acid applied 1 hr before or 1 hr after each TPA application to

28   Verma

DMBA-initiated skin inhibited skin tumor development. In contrast, if retinoic acid application was delayed as long as 24 hr post-TPA treatment,
retinoic acid did not inhibit the induction of skin tumors [19,21].

The ability to inhibit skin tumor promotion by TPA was not confined to
retinoic acid only. A number of retinoids with diverse structures were found
to inhibit skin tumor promotion by TPA. However, none of the retinoids
tested was a more potent inhibitor of tumor promotion than *trans*-retinoic
acid [19,22]. In this context, the effect of 5,6-epoxyretinoic acid (5,6-ERA)
in skin tumor promotion by TPA is noteworthy. It has been shown that
5,6-ERA may be a biologically active metabolite of retinoic acid. This conclusion is supported by the findings that 5,6-ERA detected in the intestinal
mucosa, kidney, liver, testes, and serum of vitamin A deficient rats given
[^{3}H]retinoic acid, can support growth. It is as active as *trans*-retinoic acid in
the reversal of keratinization in tracheal organ culture. We found that 5,6-
ERA is as active as retinoic acid in its ability to inhibit skin tumor promotion
by TPA [21].

The extent of inhibition of skin tumor promotion is dependent on the
duration of retinoic acid treatment [20]. We found that application of retinoic
acid, in conjunction with TPA, during the entire period (30 weeks) of the
experiment, inhibited the number of skin tumors per mouse by 82%. However, if retinoic acid application was stopped at the 10th week of promotion
treatment, and only TPA treatment was continued, the rate of skin tumor
development was the same for another 8 weeks, as was observed with mice
receiving retinoic acid treatment. Similarly, if retinoic acid application was
started at the 10th week of promotion treatment with TPA, tumor formation
was not inhibited until the 16th week of promotion treatment. Following this
delay, skin tumors developed at almost the same rate as those in groups of
mice that had received retinoic acid, in conjunction with TPA, during the
entire period of promotion treatment. These results indicate that retinoic acid
may be applied at the start of or in the later period of tumor promotion
treatments to inhibit tumor development. Gensler et al. [22] also reported the
influence of the duration of topical 13-*cis*-retinoic acid treatment on mouse
skin tumor promotion and arrived at a similar conclusion.

Certain retinoids, when administered in the diet, have been shown to
prevent and treat cancers of a variety of epithelial tissues in animal models
[17]. 13-*cis*-Retinoic acid, a geometric isomer of *trans*-retinoic acid, has
been shown to prevent chemically induced tracheobronchial cancer and urinary bladder cancer [17]. We determined the effect of dietary 13-*cis*-retinoic
acid on skin tumor promotion by TPA [24]. Dietary 13-*cis*-retinoic acid had
a major inhibitory effect on the growth of skin papillomas. In a typical
experiment with female CD-1 mice, administration of 13-*cis*-retinoic acid in
the diet was started 1 week before the first application of TPA to the DMBA-

initiated skin of these animals. Dietary 13-*cis*-retinoic acid reduced the size of skin tumors promoted with TPA; the retinoid, at doses of 5, 50, 100, 200 mg/kg of diet, inhibited the yield of papillomas (>4 mm in diameter) by 28, 55, 76, and 93%, respectively. In a separate experiment with SENCAR mice, dietary 13-*cis*-retinoic acid (100 mg/kg of diet) inhibited by 52% the incidence of carcinomas elicited by the initiation (DMBA) and promotion (TPA) protocol. Retinoid treatment did not affect body weight gains, and the survival in each experiment was more than 80% [24].

Application of nanomole quantities of retinoic acid in conjunction with TPA treatment to mouse skin inhibited the induction of ornithine decarboxylase (ODC), the key enzyme in mammalian polyamine biosynthesis [25,26]. Also, vitamin A deficient male Sprague Dawley rats showed increased ODC activity in the liver, kidney, and type II alveolar epithelial cells [27]. We observed a correlation between the ability of a specific retinoid to inhibit the induction of epidermal ODC activity and its ability to inhibit skin tumor promotion by TPA. Those retinoids that inhibited TPA-induced ODC activity, inhibited skin tumor promotion by TPA. Conversely, those retinoids that did not inhibit ODC induction, failed to inhibit tumor promotion by TPA [19]. These findings indicate that the assay for the inhibition of TPA-induced ODC by retinoids may be a simple, rapid screen for antitumor promoting properties of the new synthetic retinoids [28].

We analyzed the mechanism by which topically applied retinoic acid inhibits TPA-induced ODC activity [25,29–31]. Retinoic acid inhibition of the induction of ODC activity was not the result of nonspecific cytotoxicity, production of a soluble inhibitor of ODC, or a direct effect on the activity of ODC. In addition, inhibition of TPA-induced ODC activity was not the result of enhanced degradation and/or posttranslational modification of ODC by transglutaminase-mediated putrescine incorporation. We found that retinoic acid may inhibit TPA-induced amounts of ODC protein as determined by gel electrophoresis of immunoprecipitated difluoromethyl[^3H]ornithine-bound ODC. To obtain further clues to support the conclusion that retinoic acid may inhibit the TPA-stimulated synthesis of ODC, we determined the effect of retinoic acid on TPA-induced ODC gene expression [25]. Dot blot analysis of total cellular RNA indicates that TPA treatment resulted in an increase in the level of ODC mRNA; a peak of ODC mRNA level was observed at about 3.5 hr. 12-O-tetradecanoylphorbol-13-acetate treatment did not cause any change in the size of ODC mRNA. Northern blot analysis indicated that the epidermal RNA displayed a single major band of 2.1 kb in size either after TPA or the vehicle acetone treatment to mouse skin. Retinoic acid pretreatment restricted the increase in levels of the 2.1-kb size transcript of ODC mRNA after TPA treatment. The inhibition of ODC induction correlated with the inhibition of the induction of ODC mRNA by retinoic acid [25].

The inhibition of TPA-induced accumulation of steady-state levels of ODC mRNA may be the result either of the inhibition of transcription initiation or of the enhanced degradation of ODC mRNA. To distinguish between these two possibilities, we determined the effect of retinoic acid on the stability of ODC mRNA in the epidermal cells using pulse-chase labeling technique. In this experiment, the epidermal cells from newborn mice were pulse labeled with [^{3}H]uridine in the presence of TPA and/or TPA plus retinoic acid. At various times thereafter, cells were chased with unlabeled 5 mM uridine and 2.5 mM cytidine. Total cellular RNA was isolated and the amount of ODC mRNA was quantified by the DNA-excess filter hybridization technique [26]. The half-life of ODC mRNA, after treatment of epidermal cells with dimethyl sulfoxide (DMSO), TPA, and TPA + retinoic acid was 6.9, 7.6, and 7.9 hr, respectively. The lack of effect of TPA on the half-life of ODC mRNA indicated that TPA-induced increased steady-state levels of ODC mRNA does not result from increased ODC mRNA stability, but rather is the consequence of an increased transcription of the ODC gene. Furthermore, since retinoic acid did not affect the half-life of ODC mRNA, retinoic acid therefore does not affect the rate of degradation of ODC mRNA, but may instead inhibit TPA-induced ODC gene transcription [25].

Retinoids as Selective Chemopreventive Agents

In influencing the induction of cancer, retinoids exhibit a high degree of carcinogen, tumor promoter, and target organ specificity. A specific example is our observation that retinoic acid, applied in conjunction with TPA following initiation, inhibits the formation of skin papillomas. In contrast, retinoic acid, applied in conjunction with weekly applications of DMBA, 3-methylcholanthrene, or benzo[a]pyrene, potentiated the induction of tumors [32]. This indicates that retinoic acid, which inhibits skin tumor promotion by TPA, fails to inhibit complete carcinogenesis by the polycyclic aromatic hydrocarbons. Similarly, Gensler and Bowden [33] showed that 13-*cis*-retinoic acid does not inhibit skin tumor promotion by anthralin, a non-TPA type tumor promoter.

Further specificity of the retinoids is substantiated by the observation that 13-*cis*-retinoic acid, which inhibits urinary bladder carcinogenesis has no effect on the induction of mammary cancer in rats [17]. Similarly, dietary *N*-4-hydroxyphenyl retinamide has been shown to inhibit rat mammary carcinogenesis but paradoxically promoted mouse skin tumor formation [34]. These results indicate that the chemopreventive effects of retinoids on carcinogenesis are not universal. The mechanism underlying differential effects of retinoid remains speculative. It may be related to dose and schedule of retinoid treatment, route of administration, selective uptake and tissue deposition of a retinoid, as well as the level of retinoid acceptor and/or receptor proteins.

Retinoids as Modulators of Cell Differentiation

Retinoic acid plays an essential role in the signals that program cells for proliferation and differentiation. Hypo- and hypervitaminosis impairs the architecture and the integrity of epithelium both in animals and humans. A most dramatic effect of vitamin A deficiency is seen in tracheobronchial epithelial cells where mucous-producing columnar cells are replaced by keratinized squamous cells. Retinoic acid inhibits squamous differentiation of tracheal epithelial cells [35]. Induction of the expression of keratin 13 has been proposed to be a marker for squamous differentiation [36]. Induction of transglutaminase activity has also been associated with retinoic acid-induced differentiation of epithelial cells [37].

Besides being indispensable in maintaining normal epithelial cell morphology, retinoic acid also promotes the differentiation of carcinomal cells from a wide range of tissues [38]. Examples include differentiation of neuroblastoma cells to less malignant ganglioneurons (neuronal differentiation), teratocarcinomal cells (F9) to parietal endoderm, embryonal carcinoma cells (P19) to a variety of cell types, and hematopoietic cells (HL-60) to granulocytes [39,40]. Several mechanisms have been proposed that may be associated with retinoic acid-induced differentiation of carcinoma cells. Retinoic acid alters the expression of protooncogenes. Retinoic acid-induced differentiation of HL-60 cells to mature granulocytes is accompanied by reduction of c-myc expression [41]. Reduction of N-*myc* expression, and increased expression of the *erb B* and *src* genes correlate with growth inhibition accompanying neuronal differentiation of neuroblastoma cells [42,43]. The expression of the c-myb gene declined during maturation of neuroblastoma cells [43]. Also, a rapid decrease in phosphoinositide-derived metabolites has been implicated in the induction processes of retinoic acid-triggered neuroblastoma cell differentiation [44]. Expression of transglutaminase has been shown to be associated with cellular differentiation of human neuroblastoma cells [45]. Interestingly, secretion of laminins, glycoproteins of extracellular matrix, that have been shown to play roles in tumor progression and intercellular communication [46], is increased during differentiation of F9 cells into primitive endodermlike cells [47].

It is clear that retinoic acid-induced differentiation is accompanied by alterations in protooncogene expression, altered levels of specific keratins, basement membrane protein(s), and distinct enzymes such as transglutaminases; these observations are correlative and whether these markers are causally related to the differentiation processes is unclear.

Retinoid Binding Proteins and Nuclear Receptors as Mediators of Vitamin A Action

Vitamin A is stored as retinyl esters in the liver. Retinol is mobilized from liver stores and transported to peripheral tissues as retinol bound to a specific binding protein, serum retinol binding protein (SRBP). In the target tissue, retinol is metabolized to the aldehyde retinal, which is further oxidized irreversibly to retinoic acid [2,3]. Two specific cellular retinoid binding proteins, cellular retinol binding protein (CRBP) and cellular retinoic acid binding protein (CRABP) have been shown to exist. The CRBP and CRABP are different from the serum RBP with regard to molecular weight, immunoreactivity, and binding specificity [2]. Cellular retinol binding protein and CRABP have been completely characterized and their cDNAs have been cloned [48–50]. The role of CRBP and CRABP in mediating the action of retinoids is not unequivocally accepted. A major concern is the finding that, in hemopoietic cells (e.g., HL-60), retinoic acid is a potent inducer of differentiation but, in these cells, the CRABP and CRBP are not present at detectable levels [51,52].

A precise molecular mode of action of retinoids has not been defined. However, experimental evidence has led to two attractive hypotheses [53]. The first of these emphasizes the role of retinol as a coenzyme in the biosynthesis of membrane glycoproteins. This hypothesis is based on the observation that vitamin A deficiency causes a decrease in the incorporation of mannose into glycoproteins. In contrast, under conditions of excess vitamin A, the incorporation of mannose into liver glycoproteins is increased. The effect of vitamin A on membrane glycoprotein synthesis may be crucial because of the fact that glycoproteins, being an integral part of the plasma membrane, influence cell adhesion, growth, and cell surface properties [54].

The second hypothesis assumes that interaction of retinoic acid with the cell nucleus, mediated by specific binding protein, may lead to gene expression. For example, CRABP has been found in the nucleus [55]. As discussed earlier, vitamin A affects the expression of multiple protooncogenes such as c-myc [56]. The discovery of specific nuclear retinoic acid receptors further supports the notion that retinoids mediate their effects by modulating specific gene expression [57].

Nuclear retinoic acid receptors (RAR) belong to a superfamily of nuclear steroid–thyroid receptors [57]. However, unlike steroids, cytosolic binding proteins act as shuttles for the retinoids for the modulation of specific gene transcription [55,58]. The cDNAs encoding putative nuclear retinoic acid receptors have been cloned and characterized. At least three (α, β, γ) distinct subtypes of nuclear retinoic acid receptor, from both mouse and human, have been identified [57–62]. There is a remarkable amino acid sequence homology between mouse and human RARs. The RAR subtypes are expressed differentially in various tissues. The RARα gene is expressed in hematopoietic tissues while RARγ is predominantly expressed in skin [61]. The RARβ gene is induced in response to retinoic acid and appears to be regulated at the transcriptional level. The half-life of RARβ mRNA is short (~50 min), however, RARα and RARγ genes are not inducible and are expressed from relatively stable mRNA ($t^{1/2}$ to ~5 hr) [63]. The RARα gene was mapped to chromosome 17q21 and the gene for RARβ was mapped to chromosome 3p21-25 [64]. The functional retinoic acid responsive element (RARE) in the β gene that mediates trans-activation of the gene by retinoic acid has been identified as a 27 base pair sequence, located 59 base pairs upstream of the transcriptional start [63]. Recently, a similar RARE in the 5′-flanking region of the laminin B1 gene has been identified [47].

The biological significance of differential expression of retinoic acid nuclear receptors in various tissues has not been defined. Recent findings [65] indicate that the level of nuclear RARs may not be crucial in retinoic acid-induced differentiation of HL-60 cells. Also, there is little information about the level, nature, and regulation of nuclear RAR proteins. Further research about the nuclear RAR proteins and their responsive elements in transcriptionally regulated genes will advance our knowledge about the mechanism of action of retinoids.

SUMMARY AND CONCLUSIONS

Vitamin A (retinol), in humans, is essential for the maintenance of growth, reproduction, and vision. Retinoic acid, a major metabolite of circulating retinol, is essential to maintain the normal pathway of differentiation of epithelial tissues but cannot support the visual and reproductive functions of retinol. Vitamin A deficiency results in susceptibility to carcinogenesis. Certain retinoids inhibit the induction of cancer in experimental animals but exhibit a high degree of target organ specificity. Retinoids have also been used in the prevention [66] and treatment of human cancer [67] but the oral use of the retinoids is handicapped by their toxic side-effects [68]. Retinoic acid promotes differentiation of certain carcinoma cells and also inhibits the proliferation of certain tumor cell lines. The molecular basis of this retinoid action is not yet defined. Retinoids modulate the expression of specific protooncogenes, peptide growth factors [16], and also influence the host immune system [69].

ACKNOWLEDGMENTS

The work was supported in part by United States Public Health Service Grant CA-42585 by the National Cancer Institute.

REFERENCES

1. Dowling JE, Wald G (1980): The biological function of vitamin A acid. Proc Natl Acad Sci USA 46:587–608.
2. Goodman DS (1979): Vitamin A metabolism. Fed Proc 38:2716–2722.
3. DeLuca HF (1979): Retinoic acid metabolism. Fed Proc 38:2519–2523.
4. Favennec L, Cals MJ (1988): The biological effects of retinoids on cell differentiation and proliferation. J Clin Chem Clin Biochem 26:479–489.
5. Brickell PM, Tickle C (1989): Morphogens in chick limb development. Bioessays 11: 145–149.
6. De Luca LM, Roop D, Huang FL (1985): Vitamin A: a key nutrient for the maintenance of epithelial differentiation. Acta Vitaminal Enzymol 7:13–20.
7. Middleton B, Byers T, Marshall J, Graham S (1986): Dietary vitamin A and cancer—a multisite case-control study. Nutr Cancer 8:107–116.
8. Hinds MW, Kolonel LN, Hankin JH, Lee J (1984): Dietary vitamin A, carotene, vitamin C and risk of lung cancer in Hawaii. Am J Epidemiol 119:227–237.
9. Mettlin C, Graham S, Swanson M (1979): Vitamin A and lung cancer. J Natl Cancer Inst 62:1435–1438.
10. Connett JE, Kuller LH, Kjelsberg MO, Polk BF, Collins G, Rider A, Hulley SB (1989): Relationship between carotenoids and cancer. Cancer 64:126–134.
11. Narisawa T, Reddy BS, Wong CQ, Weisburger JH (1976): Effect of vitamin A deficiency on rat colon carcinogenesis by N-methyl-N'-nitro-N-nitrosoguanidine. Cancer Res 36: 1379–1383.
12. Nettesheim P, Williams ML (1976): The influence of vitamin A on the susceptibility of the rat lung to 3-methylcholanthrene. Int J Cancer 17:351–357.
13. Boutwell RK (1974): The function and mechanism of promoters of carcinogenesis. CRC Crit Rev Toxicol 2:419–443.
14. Verma AK, Boutwell RK (1980): Effects of dose and duration of treatment with the tumor promoting agent 12-O-tetradecanoylphorbol-13-acetate on mouse skin carcinogenesis. Carcinogenesis 1:271–276.
15. Verma AK (1985): Mouse skin carcinogenesis. In Maihach HI, Lowe NJ (eds): "Models in Dermatology," New York: Karger, Vol 2, pp 313–321.
16. Bertram JS, Kolonel LN, Meyskens FL (1987): Rationale and strategies for chemoprevention of cancer in humans. Cancer Res 47:3012–3031.
17. Moon RC, McCormick DL, Mehta RG (1983): Inhibition of carcinogenesis by retinoids. Cancer Res 43:2469–2475.
18. Sporn MB, Roberts AB (1983): Role of retinoids in differentiation and carcinogenesis. Cancer Res 43:3034–3040.
19. Verma AK, Shapas BG, Rice HM, Boutwell RK (1979): Correlation of the inhibition by retinoids of tumor promoter-induced mouse epidermal ornithine decarboxylase activity and of skin tumor promotion. Cancer Res 39:419–425.
20. Verma AK (1987): Inhibition of both stage I and stage II mouse skin tumor promotion by retinoic acid and the dependence of inhibition of tumor promotion on the duration of retinoic acid treatment. Cancer Res 47:5097–5101.
21. Verma AK, Slaga TJ, Wertz PW, Mueller GC, Boutwell RK (1980): Inhibition of skin tumor promotion by retinoic acid and its metabolite 5,6-epoxyretinoic acid. Cancer Res 40:2367–2371.
22. Verma AK, Boutwell RK (1977): Vitamin A acid (retinoic acid), a potent inhibitor of 12-O-tetradecanoyl-phorbol-13-acetate-induced ornithine decarboxylase activity in mouse epidermis. Cancer Res 37:2196–2201.

23. Gensler HL, Sim DA, Bowden GT (1986): Influence of the duration of topical 13-*cis*-retinoic acid treatment on inhibition of mouse skin tumor promotion. Cancer Res 46:2767–2770.

24. Verma AK, Duvick L, Ali M (1986): Modulation of mouse skin tumor promotion by dietary 13-*cis*-retinoic acid and alpha difluoromethylornithine. Carcinogenesis 7:1019–1023.

25. Verma AK (1988): Inhibition of tumor promoter 12-O-tetradecanoylphorbol-13-acetate-induced synthesis of epidermal ornithine decarboxylase messenger RNA and diacylglycerol-promoted mouse skin tumor formation by retinoic acid. Cancer Res 48:2168–2173.

26. Hsieh JT, Denning MF, Heidel SM, Verma AK (1990): Expression of human chromosome 2 ornithine decarboxylase gene in ornithine decarboxylase-deficient chinese hamster ovary cell. Cancer Res 50:2239–2244.

27. Verma AK, Zatchman RD, Simsiman R, Shoemaker A, Menning M (1990): Correlation between retinoic acid nuclear receptor gene expression and increased ornithine decarboxylase activity in the kidney and liver of vitamin A deficient rats. Proc Am Assoc Cancer Res 31:127.

28. Verma AK, Rice HM, Shapas BG, Boutwell RK (1978): Inhibition of 12-O-tetradecanoylphorbol-13-acetate-induced ornithine decarboxylase activity in mouse epidermis by vitamin A analog (retinoids). Cancer Res 38:793–801.

29. Verma AK (1985): Inhibition of phorbol ester-caused synthesis of mouse epidermal ornithine decarboxylase by retinoic acid. Biochim Biophys Acta 846:109–119.

30. Verma AK, Erickson D, Dolnick BJ (1986): Increased mouse epidermal ornithine decarboxylase activity by the tumor promoter 12-O-tetradecanoylphorbol-13-acetate involves increased amounts of both enzyme protein and messenger RNA. Biochem J 237:297–300.

31. Verma AK, Pong RC, Erickson D (1986): Involvement of protein kinase C activation in ornithine decarboxylase gene expression in primary culture of newborn mouse epidermal cells and in skin tumor promotion by 12-O-tetradecanoylphorbol-13-acetate. Cancer Res 46:6149–6155.

32. Verma AK, Conrad EA, Boutwell RK (1982): Differential effects of retinoic acid and 7,8-benzoflavone on the induction of mouse skin tumors by the complete carcinogenesis process and by the initiation-promotion regimen. Cancer Res 42:3519–3525.

33. Gensler H, Bowden GT (1984): Influence of 13-*cis*-retinoic acid treatment on inhibition of mouse skin tumor promotion. Cancer Lett 22:71–75.

34. McCormick DL, Bagg BJ, Hultin TA (1987): Comparative activity of dietary or topical exposure to three retinoids in the promotion of skin tumor induction in mice. Cancer Res 47:5989–5993.

35. Clark JN, Marchok AC (1979): The effect of vitamin A on cellular differentiation and mucous glycoprotein synthesis in long-term rat tracheal organ cultures. Differentiation 14:175–183.

36. Jetten AM, George MA, Smits HL, Vollberg TM (1989): Keratin 13 expression is linked to squamous differentiation in rabbit tracheal epithelial cells and down-regulated by retinoic acid. Exp Cell Res 182:622–634.

37. Lichti U, Yuspa SH (1988): Modulation of tissue epidermal transglutaminase in mouse epidermal cells after treatment with 12-O-tetredecanoylphorbol-13-acetate in vivo and in culture. Cancer Res 48:74–81.

38. Jetten AM, Jetten ME, Sherman MI (1979): Stimulation of differentiation of several murine embryonal carcinoma cell lines by retinoic acid. Exp Cell Res 124:381–391.

39. Imaizumi M, Breitman TR (1987): Retinoic acid-induced differentiation of the human promyelocytic leukemia cell line, HL-60, and fresh human leukemia cells in primary

culture: a model for differentiation inducing therapy of leukemia. Eur J Haematol 38: 289–302.

40. Miki K, Kitagawa Y (1988): Biphasic response to retinoic acid dose in differentiation of F9 cells into primitive endoderm-like cells. Exp Cell Res 179:344–351.

41. Bentley DL, Groudine M (1986): A block to elongation is largely responsible for decreased transcription of c-myc in differentiated HL 60 cells. Nature (London) 321:702–706.

42. Thiele CJ, Deutsch LA, Israel MA (1988): The expression of multiple protooncogenes is differentially regulated during retinoic acid-induced maturation of human neuroblastoma cell lines. Oncogene 3:281–288.

43. Thiele CJ, Cohen PS, Israel MA (1988): Regulation of c-myb expression in human neuroblastoma cells during retinoic acid-induced differentiation. Mol Cell Biol 8:1677–1683.

44. Lanciotti M, Longone P, Cornaglia-Ferraris P, Ponzoni M (1989): Retinoic acid inhibits phosphatidylinositol turnover only in RA-sensitive while not in RA-resistant human neuroblastoma cells. Biochem Biophys Res Commun 161:284–289.

45. Melino G, Farrace MG, Ceru MP, Piacentini M (1988): Correlation between transglutaminase activity and polyamine levels in human neuroblastoma cells. Effect of retinoic acid and alpha-difluoromethylornithine. Exp Cell Res 179:429–445.

46. Beck K, Hunter I, Engel J (1990): Structure and function of laminin: anatomy of a multidomain glycoprotein. FASEB J. 4:148–160.

47. Vasios GW, Gold JD, Petkovich M, Chambon P, Gudas LJ (1989): A retinoic acid-responsive element is present in the 5' flanking region of the laminin B1 gene. Proc Natl Acad Sci USA 86:9099–9103.

48. Ong DE, Crow JA, Chytil F (1982): Radioimmunochemical determination of cellular retinol- and cellular retinoic acid-binding proteins in cytosols of rat tissues. J Biol Chem 257:13385–13389.

49. Blaner WS (1989): Retinol-binding protein. the serum transport protein for vitamin A. Endo Rev 10:308–315.

50. Shubeita HE, Sambrook JF, McCormick AM (1987): Molecular cloning and analysis of functional cDNA and genomic clones encoding bovine cellular retinoic acid-binding protein. Proc Natl Acad Sci USA 84:5648–5649.

51. Jetten AM, Anderson K, Deas MA, Kagechika H, Lotan R, Rearick JI, Shudo K (1987): New benzoic acid derivatives with retinoid activity: lack of direct correlation between biological activity and binding to cellular retinoic acid binding protein. Cancer Res 47: 3523–3527.

52. Nervi C, Grippo JF, Sherman MI, George MD, Jetten AM (1989): Identification and characterization of nuclear retinoic acid-binding activity in human myeloblastic leukemia HL-60 cells. Proc Natl Acad Sci USA 86:5854–5858.

53. Omori M, Chytil F (1982): Mechanism of vitamin A action: gene expression in retinol-deficient rats. J Biol Chem 257:14370–14374.

54. Creek KE, Rimoldi D, Silverman-Jones CS, DeLuca LM (1985): Synthesis of retinyl phosphate mannose in vitro: non-enzymatic breakdown and reversibility. Biochem J 227: 695–703.

55. Sani BP (1977): Localization of retinoic acid binding protein in nuclei. Biochem Biophys Res Commun 75:7–12.

56. Nakamura KD, Hart RW (1989): Proto-oncogene expression during retinoic acid-induced neural differentiation of embryonal carcinoma cells. Mech Ageing Dev 48:53–62.

57. Petkovich M, Brand N, Krust J, Chambon P (1987): A human retinoic acid receptor which belongs to the family of nuclear receptors. Nature (London) 330:444–450.

58. Takase S, Ong DE, Chytil F (1987): Transfer of retinoic acid from its complex with cellular retinoic acid-binding protein to the nucleus. Arch Biochem Biophys 247:328–334.
59. Brand N, Petkovich M, Krust A, Chambon P, de The H, Marchio A, Tiollais P, Dejean A (1988): Identification of a second human retinoic acid receptor. Nature 332:850–853.
60. Benbrook D, Lernhardt E, Pfahl M (1988): A new retinoic acid receptor identified from a hepatocellular carcinoma. Nature 333:669–672.
61. Zelent A, Krust A, Petkovich M, Kastner P, Chambon P (1989): Cloning of murine alpha and beta retinoic acid receptors and a novel receptor gamma predominately expressed in skin. Nature 339:714–717.
62. Krust A, Kastner P, Petkovich M, Zelent A, Chambon P (1989): A third human retinoic acid receptor, hRAR-gamma. Proc Natl Acad Sci USA 86:5310–5314.
63. de The H, Vivanco-Ruiz M, del M, Tiollais P, Stunneneberg H, Dejean A (1990): Identification of a retinoic acid responsive element in the retinoic acid receptor beta gene. Nature 343:177–180.
64. Mattei MG, de The H, Mattei JF, Marchio A, Tiollais P, Dejean A (1988): Assignment of the human hap retinoic acid receptor RAR beta gene to the p24 band of chromosome 3. Hum Genet 80:189–190.
65. Wang C, Curtis JE, Minden MD, McCulloch EA (1989): Expression of a retinoic acid receptor gene in myeloid leukemia cells. Leukemia 3:264–269.
66. Lippman SM, Meyskens FL (1988): Vitamin A derivatives in the prevention and treatment of human cancer. J Am Coll Nutr 7:269–284.
67. Orfanos CE, Ehlert R, Gollnick H (1987): The retinoids. A review of their clinical pharmacology and therapeutic use. Drugs 34:459–503.
68. David M, Hodak E, Lowe NJ (1988): Adverse effects of retinoids. Med Toxicol Adverse Drug Exp 3:273–288.
69. Dennert G (1985): Immunostimulation by retinoic acid. Ciba Found Symp 113:117–131.

Vitamins and Cancer Prevention, pages 39–49
© *1991 Wiley-Liss, Inc.*

4 | Localized Folate Deficiency and Cancer

Carlos L. Krumdieck, M.D., Ph.D.

In 1973, Whitehead, Reyner and Lindenbaum [1] published a seminal article describing the presence of megaloblastic changes in cervical epithelial cells from women who were using steroid hormones as oral contraceptive agents (OCA). As many as 19% of the OCA users showed cytological abnormalities which, although not associated with systemic evidence of folate or B_{12} deficiency, were corrected by the administration of oral folic acid. The authors postulated that a localized deficiency of folates in the cervix had developed as a result of OCA use. Three years later our laboratory showed that the folate content of the uterus is indeed influenced by variations in the levels of sex hormones, demonstrating cyclical changes in the concentration of uterine folates during the estrus cycle in rats [2,3].

The possible association of localized folate deficiency, brought about by OCA use, with preoplastic lesions of cervical dysplasia, was envisioned by Butterworth [4] based on the morphological similarity of folate-deficient epithelial cells and the cells observed in cervical dysplasia [5]. In 1982, Butterworth [4] postulated that ''. . . chronic exposure of target tissues to contraceptive steroids might produce localized alterations in folic acid metabolism in such a way as to favor neoplastic transformation.'' These authors attempted to correct the putative localized deficiency by exogenous supplementation of the vitamin to see if it was possible to alter the course of early cervical dysplasia. Under double-blind conditions, 47 women users of OCA,

Department of Nutrition Sciences, University of Alabama at Birmingham, Birmingham, Alabama 35294

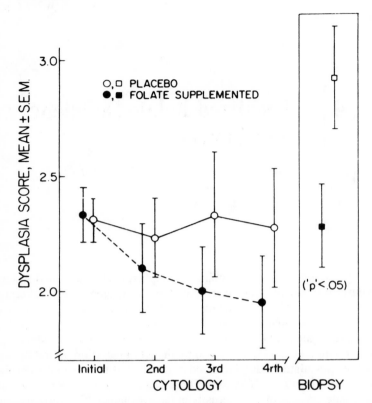

Fig. 1.   Cervical dysplasia scores (mean ± SEM) showing successive changes from the first visit at which time the protocol was initiated with daily oral doses of either folic acid or placebo. Follow-up smears were obtained at monthly intervals. Reprinted with permission from Butterworth et al. Am J Clin Nutr 35:73–82 (1982). Copyright © Am J Clin Nutr, American Society for Clinical Nutrition.

diagnosed as having mild or moderate cervical dysplasia by cervical smears, received either 10 mg of folic acid per day or a placebo for 3 months. Papanicolaou smears obtained once a month and a biopsy taken at the end of the study were evaluated blindly by a single pathologist using the following scoring system: 1 normal, 2 mild, 3 moderate, 4 severe, and 5 carcinoma in situ. The results are summarized in Fig. 1. At the outset, the pretreatment scores of the two treatment groups were very similar. For patients receiving folate, their final cytology score was significantly improved, compared to their initial score (paired t test; $p < 0.05$), while in the placebo-treated group their cytology scores were unchanged. The biopsy scores were also significantly lower in folate-supplemented subjects than in placebo subjects (2.28

TABLE I. Cervical Dysplasia. Rate of Regression to Normal

Reference		Rate	0/00
7		From mild	$6/462 \approx 13$
		From moderate	$0/462 \approx 0$
6		Severity not specified	$0/93 \approx 0$
4	Placebo	From Mild	$1/25 \approx 50$
		From Moderate	0/25
	Folate	From mild	$1/22 \approx 40$
		From moderate	$4/22 \approx 200$

TABLE II. Cervical Dysplasia. Rate of Progression to Carcinoma In Situ

Reference		(‰ /year)
8		106
7		160
4	Placebo	$4/25 \approx 160$
	Folate	0/22

$\pm$ 0.19 vs 2.92 $\pm$ 0.22; mean $\pm$ SEM; $p < 0.05$ unpaired t test) indicating again a beneficial effect of the supplements. The rates of regression to normal and of progression to carcinoma in situ that were observed in this study were compared to those reported in the literature documenting the natural course of dysplasia in the absence of therapy [6–8] and are summarized in Tables I and II. In our study, folate supplementation produced regression of moderate dysplasia to normal in four cases, a phenomenon never previously observed in untreated cases (Table I). Equally as important, 4 of the 25 subjects on placebo progressed to carcinoma in situ while none among the 22 supplemented subjects did so (Table II). The results of this study indicated that morphological manifestations of dysplasia improved after 3 months of folic acid supplementation while remaining stable or progressing in nonsupplemented controls.

These findings stimulated us to look for a different human model of localized folate deficiency associated with preneoplastic lesions that could be used to confirm the above results.

The idea to use smokers with bronchial metaplasia was originally conceived on the basis of studies demonstrating that cyanide intake associated with cigarette smoking [9] adversely affects B_{12} nutritional status [10,11]. Urine thiocyanate excretion, which is an index of the exogenous cyanide load, correlates negatively with serum B_{12} concentrations, and positively with urinary B_{12} excretion. The cyanides readily combine with hydroxocobalamin to form cyanocobalamin, which is inactive as a coenzyme form of the vitamin and is usually undetectable in tissues. In contrast, in subjects

TABLE III. Plasma and RBC Folate Levels in Nonsmokers and in Smokers With and Without Bronchial Metaplasia*

Group	Plasma FA (ng/ml)	RBC FA (ng/ml)
Nonsmokers	8.0 ± 1.0^{abc}	322 ± 27^{efg}
All smokers	5.5 ± 0.4^{a}	261 ± 13^{e}
Smokers without metaplasia	6.3 ± 0.6^{bd}	277 ± 18^{fh}
Smokers with metaplasia	4.9 ± 0.5^{cd}	251 ± 17^{gh}
Class 1	5.7 ± 1.9	264 ± 38
Class 2	5.0 ± 0.7	261 ± 24
Class 3–4	4.8 ± 0.8	235 ± 33

*Levels are means $\pm$ SEM. FA = folic acid; RBC = red blood cell. Pairs of values with the same superscript letters are compared statistically by the Wilcoxon rank-sum test, with p values as follows: a,p = 0.02; b,f,h, p = >0.05; c,p = 0.004; d,p = 0.03; e,p = 0.04; g, p = 0.03.

suffering from tobacco amblyopia, plasma levels of cyanocobalamins increase markedly from a normal value of less than 8% of total cobalamins to as much as 35%. In addition to the detrimental effect of hydrogen cyanide on B_{12} nutritional status, hydrogen sulfide, which is also present in the gas phase of cigarette smoke [9] has an even greater affinity for the corrin cobalt than the CN- group of cyanides. Moreover, nitrous oxide (N_2O) is also present in the cigarette smoke; this gas can inactivate methylcobalamin through oxidation of the cobalt atom [12] and, in addition, irreversibly inactivate the methylcobalamin-requiring enzyme methionine synthetase [13]. We reasoned that if tobacco smoke lowered systemic levels of B_{12} in a dose-related fashion, it might have an even greater impact on the B_{12} content of the lung epithelia, which is clearly the tissue most proximately exposed to the deleterious effects of the smoke. We predicted that a folate deficiency secondary to the now unequivocally established methyl folate trap [14] should develop in the B_{12}-depleted epithelia of the smokers. In addition to our postulated B_{12}-mediated mechanism of production of localized folate deficiency in smokers, a number of other mechanisms resulting from various reactions of smoke components directly with tetrahydrofolates may contribute to the in situ inactivation of these cofactors. These include the reaction of tetrahydrofolates with cyanates (or their reactive form isocyanic acid) to form a biologically inactive derivative [15] and the reaction of methyltetrahydrofolates with organic nitrites leading to decomposition of the coenzymes [16]. It should also be noted that organic nitrites can inactivate methylcobalamin by cleaving the methyl–Co bond with the ultimate formation of nitrocobalamin [16].

It has been demonstrated by Witter et al. [17], Nakazawa et al. [18], and by our own studies [19] (Table III) that the mechanisms described above, and

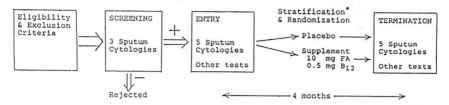

Fig. 2. Randomized Double-Blind Folate/B_{12} Supplementation of Smokers with Bronchial Metaplasia. (*) Stratification by smoking level.

TABLE IV. Criteria for Eligibility and Exclusion

Criteria Of	
Eligibility	Exclusion
≥20 pack-years smoking	FA/B_{12} supplementation > RDA
Currently smoking	FA/B_{12} deficiency
Metaplasia on ≥1 sample	Marijuana or anticonvulsant use
	Lung cancer
	Intestinal pathology
	Alcohol abuse

very possibly others, can indeed adversely affect folate nutritional status. All of these studies showed significantly lower circulating levels of folates in smokers.

With this background information, we decided to carry out an intervention trial, of similar design to the cervical dysplasia study, to test whether preneoplastic lesions in chronic smokers could be improved by supplements of folic acid and vitamin B_{12} [20]. A double-blind, randomized, prospective trial was designed as shown in Fig. 2. Subjects with diagnosed squamous metaplasia were recruited from a previously identified population of 9400 male cigarette smokers who had been screened in 1973 for the Multiple Risk Factor Intervention Trial for prevention of coronary disease. The criteria for eligibility and exclusion are listed in Table IV. The diagnosis of squamous metaplasia was made by sputum cytology. At screening, three deep-cough sputum samples were examined and a positive diagnosis made if any of them showed squamous metaplasia. Subsequently, the baseline scoring of the metaplasia was established from five new sputum samples obtained at entry into the study. Cytological evaluation of these specimens was performed initially according to the standard criteria of the International Histological Classification of Tumors [21]. All samples were evaluated by a single cytopathologist. The severity of the lesions were scored as follows: 0, normal cytology, satisfactory specimen (pulmonary alveolar macrophages present, signs of acute infection absent); 1, squamous metaplasia without atypia; 2, squamous metaplasia with mild atypia; 3, squamous metaplasia with moderate atypia; and 4, squamous metaplasia with severe atypia. The worst score of the five samples was used in analysis. Following determination of circulating levels of folate, B_{12} and other vitamins, and of the numbers of cigarettes consumed per day (all repeated at termination), the subjects were randomly assigned to either the placebo or treatment groups. Identical opaque capsules, containing either lactose or 10 mg of folic acid plus 0.5 mg of hydroxocobalamin, were distributed to the respective groups and the subjects were instructed to take one capsule per day. Compliance was monitored by monthly telephone calls. After 4 months, the subjects returned and another five sputum samples were evaluated for squamous metaplasia as described above. Seventy-three subjects (37 on placebo and 36 on supplement) completed the 4 month study. Because only 8 of the 73 subjects had cytology scores of 3 or 4 at entry or termination, scores 2, 3, and 4 were combined to include all subjects with atypia and an abridged scoring system was finally used: 0, normal cytology–satisfactory specimen; 1, squamous metaplasia without atypia; and 2, squamous metaplasia with atypia (mild, moderate, or severe). A reduction or an increase in score of at least one point was taken to indicate improvement or worsening, respectively; all others were considered unchanged. We found that more subjects receiving the supplement exhibited improvement and fewer got worse compared to those receiving the placebo (Fig. 3). Table V is a transition matrix comparing the supplement and placebo groups directly. The numbers in parentheses indicate the number of transitions in cytology expected in the supplemented group (calculated from those observed in the placebo group) if the supplement had no effect. The supplement group improved significantly compared to the placebo group (p = 0.02). The predominant contribution to the significance of this test is from subjects who had atypia at entry and not at termination. Thus, it seems that the supplement reduced the prevalence of atypia but not that of squamous metaplasia. Tables VI and VII compare the transitions observed in the placebo and supplement groups with those expected (numbers in parentheses) calculated from the estimate of random variation in cytology scores observed in the entire study population during the nonintervention period that elapsed between screening and entry. Table VI shows, as expected, that subjects on placebo showed no change during the trial compared to random variation (p = 0.2), while the supplemented subjects (Table VII) improved significantly compared to random variation (p = 0.0002).

The results of this trial, using a different model of "localized" folate deficiency, are in agreement with those of the previous cervical dysplasia study but do not remove a number of important limitations, applying to both studies, that must be kept in mind when interpreting these findings. Perhaps the most important caveat is that the folate–B_{12}-dependent *morphological*

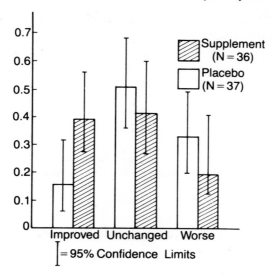

0.7 ┤

0.6 ┤   ▨ Supplement
                (N = 36)
0.5 ┤   ☐ Placebo
                (N = 37)
0.4 ┤

0.3 ┤

0.2 ┤

0.1 ┤

0 ┴──────────────────────────
   Improved Unchanged Worse

I = 95% Confidence Limits

Fig. 3. Proportion of patients that improved, remained the same, and worsened on placebo ☐ (N = 37) and supplement ▨ (N = 36). Vertical bars, which represent 95% confidence intervals, are unrelated to primary statistical test applied to data (chi-square). Reprinted with permission from Heimburger et al. J Am Med Assoc 259:1525–1530 (1988). Copyright © 1988, American Medical Association.

TABLE V. Observed and (Expected)[a] Cytology Score Transitions From Entry to Termination in Subjects on Supplement Compared to Subjects on Placebo[b]

	Cytology score	Study termination		
		0	1	2
	0	7	0	7
		(6.3)	(3.5)	(4.2)
Study	1	3	2	0
entry		(2)	(2)	(1)
	2	2	9	6
		(1.4)	(4.3)	(11.4)

[a]Calculated from results in Placebo group. Shaded area indicates no change; above shaded area, worsened; below, improved.
[b]Improvement on supplement versus placebo.
$X^2_6 = 14.9$ $p = 0.02$

improvements in cervical dysplasia scores and in squamous metaplasia with atypia cannot be taken as conclusive evidence indicative of a reduction of cancer risk. We still do not know if the morphological lesions of folate deficiency and of cervical dysplasia or squamous metaplasia with atypia, although indistinguishable by present methods, correspond to completely

TABLE VI. Observed and (Expected)[a] Cytology Score Transitions From Entry to Termination. Placebo Group[b]

	Cytology score	Study termination		
		0	1	2
Study entry	0	9 (8.4)	5 (3.9)	6 (7.7)
	1	2 (1.5)	2 (1.5)	1 (1.9)
	2	1 (5.5)	3 (1.8)	8 (4.6)

[a]Calculated from variation in pretrial period. Shaded area indicates no change; above shaded area, worsened; below, improved.
[b]No difference between placebo and random variation.
$X^2_6 = 8.5$ $p = 0.2$

TABLE VII. Observed and (Expected)[a] Cytology Score Transitions From Entry to Termination. Supplement Group

	Cytology score	Study termination		
		0	1	2
Study entry	0	7 (5.9)	0 (2.7)	7 (5.4)
	1	3 (1.5)	2 (1.5)	0 (2.0)
	2	2 (7.8)	9 (2.6)	6 (6.5)

Improvement on supplement versus random variation: $X^2_6 = 26.9$ $p = 0.0002$
[a]Calculated from variation in pretrial period. Shaded area indicates no change; above shaded area, worsened; below, improved.

unrelated processes, the former benign and the latter two potentially malignant. Morphologically identical benign manifestations of vitamin deficiency may therefore be misdiagnosed as preneoplastic lesions. This question will remain unresolved until conclusive evidence is obtained that folate-deficient cells are (or are not) indeed more susceptible to neoplastic transformation and that they should (or should not) be considered as an early (reversible) stage in the progression to cancer.

Another important limitation of studies to this date is that the postulated states of localized deficiency, although supported by strong indirect evidence, have not been unequivocally demonstrated by the direct determination of vitamin levels in the affected tissues.

We attempted to resolve this issue by analyzing the total folate content of biopsy specimens obtained from patients undergoing bronchoscopy for medically indicated reasons. We chose as the biopsy site the carina tracheae because of the minimal risk associated with biopsies of this site, and in order

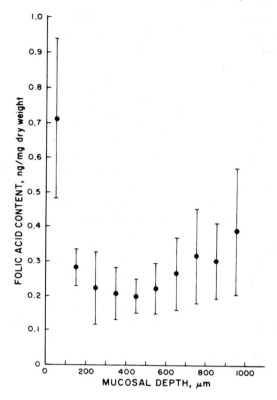

Fig. 4. Total folate content (*L. casei* assay) of six serially sliced dog tracheas (mean ± SD). Reprinted with permission from Heim et al. J Am Med Assoc 259:1525–1530 (1988). Copyright © 1988, American Medical Association.

to minimize possible variations in folate content that might occur with samples obtained from various parts of the bronchial tree. Folate concentrations were higher in the smaller biopsy specimens with samples greater than 1 mg of dry weight (n = 10) having a folate content (mean ± SEM) of 0.309 ± 0.061 ng/mg and samples smaller than 1 mg (N = 6) having 0.56 ± 0.097 ng of folate/mg (p < 0.05 by Student's t test). We attributed this to an uneven distribution of folates in the mucosal and submucosal layers of the epithelium with the former, predominating in the smaller samples, having a higher folate content. This assumption was verified by analyzing the folate content of microtome slices of dog trachea cut parallel to the surface of the epithelium in 100 μm increments. The most superficial 100 μm slice indeed had a markedly higher folate content (Fig. 4) [19]. Clearly, if this observation is also true for humans, results obtained by analyzing human biopsy specimens for folate levels will vary unpredictably unless one can restrict the sampling to the outermost layer(s) of the epithelium.

Progress in the study of the role of localized folate deficiency in carcinogenesis has been severely hampered by the lack of an animal model in which it could be unequivocally demonstrated that the deficient cells progress to cancer upon carcinogen exposure. A suitable model may be developed taking advantage of the observation that mature circulating unstimulated human lymphocytes do not incorporate appreciable amounts of folate from the extracellular medium [22]. As a result, lymphocytes can continue to exhibit evidence of folate deficiency for periods of up to 3 months after correction of a deficiency state by appropriate therapy. If this phenomenon can be observed in an animal susceptible to the production of severe folate deficiency such as the guinea pig [23], it may be possible, by acute correction of a severe folate deficiency, to establish for a limited time a situation of folate deficiency "localized" to the mature lymphocytes. These cells are readily sampled, permitting direct estimation of the severity of the localized deficiency. Moreover, stimulation of proliferation of this folate-deficient cell cohort by antigenic challenge may serve as a promoter stimulus, much as partial hepatectomy is used in experimental liver-cancer production. Much additional research obviously lies ahead before the hypothesis that localized folate and/or B_{12} deficiencies can render the affected tissues more susceptible to neoplastic transformation is either proven or disproven.

REFERENCES

1. Whitehead N, Reyner F, Lindenbaum J (1973): Megaloblastic changes in the cervical epithelium: Association with oral contraceptive therapy and reversal with folic acid. J Am Med Assoc 226:1421–1424.
2. Krumdieck CL, Boots LR, Cornwell PE, Butterworth CE Jr (1975): Estrogen stimulation of conjugase activity in the uterus of ovariectomized rats. Am J Clin Nutr 28:530–534.
3. Krumdieck CL, Boots LR, Cornwell PE, Butterworth CE, Jr (1976): Cyclic variations in folate composition and pteroyl polyglutamyl hydrolase (conjugase) activity of the rat uterus. Am J Clin Nutr 29:288–294.
4. Butterworth CE Jr, Hatch KD, Gore H, Mueller H, Krumdieck CL (1982): Improvement in cervical dysplasia associated with folic acid therapy in users of oral contraceptives. Am J Clin Nutr 35:73–82.
5. Koss LG (1979): Diagnostic Cytology and its Histopathic Bases 3rd ed. Philadelphia: Lippincott.
6. Koss LG et al. (1963): Some histological aspects of behavior of epidermoid carcinoma in situ and related lesions of the uterine cervix. Cancer 16:1160.
7. Richart RM, Barron BA (1969): A follow-up study of patients with cervical dysplasia. Am J Obstet Gynecol 105:386.
8. Stern E, Neely PM (1963): Carcinoma and dysplasia of the cervix: A comparison of rates for new and returning populations. Acta Cytol 7:357.

9. Stedman RL (1968): The chemical composition of tobacco and tobacco smoke. Chem Rev 68:153–207.
10. Linnell JC, Smith ADM, Smith CL, Wilson J, Matthews DM (1968): Effects of smoking on metabolism and excretion of vitamin B_{12}. Br Med J 27:215–216.
11. Dastur DK, Quadros EV, Wadia NH, Desai MM, Bharucha EP (1972): Effect of vegetarianism and smoking on vitamin B_{12}, thiocyanate, and folate levels in the blood of normal subjects. Br Med J 29:260–263.
12. Kondo H, Osborne ML, Kolhouse JF, Binder MJ, Podell ER, Utley CS, Abrams RS, Allen RH (1981): Nitrous oxide has multiple deleterious effects on cobalamin metabolism and causes decreases in activities of both mammalian cobalamin-dependent enzymes in rats. J Clin Invest 67:1270–1283.
13. Frasca V, Riazzi BS, Matthews RG (1986): In vitro inactivation of methionine synthase by nitrous oxide. J Biol Chem 5:261(34):15823–15826.
14. Fujii K, Nagasaki T, Vitols KS, Huennekens FM (1983): Polyglutamylation as a factor in the trapping of 5-methyltetrahydrofolate by cobalamin-deficient L1210 cells. In Bertino JR (eds): "Folyl and antifolyl polyglutamates." New York; Plenum, pp 375–397.
15. Francis KT, Thompson RW, Krumdieck CL (1977): Reaction of tetrahydrofolic acid with cyanate from urea solutions: formation of an inactive folate derivative. Am J Clin Nutr 30:2028–2032.
16. Khaled MA, Watkins CL, Krumdieck CL (1986): Inactivation of B12 and folate coenzymes by butyl nitrite as observed by NMR: Implications on one-carbon transfer mechanisms. Biochem Biophys Res Commun 135:201–207.
17. Witter FR, Blake DA, Baumgardner R, Mellits ED, Niebyl JR (1982): Folate, carotene, and smoking. Am J Obstet Gynecol 144:857.
18. Nakazawa Y, Chiba K, Imatoh N, Kotorii T, Sakamoto T, Ishizaki T (1983): Serum folic acid levels and antipyrine clearance rates in smokers and non-smokers. Drug Alcohol Dep 11:201.
19. Heimburger DC, Krumdieck CL, Alexander CB, Birch R, Dill SR, Bailey WC (1987): Localized folic acid deficiency and bronchial metaplasia in smokers: Hypothesis and preliminary report. Nutr Int 3:54–60.
20. Heimburger DC, Alexander CB, Birch R, Butterworth CE, Jr, Bailey WC, Krumdieck CL (1988): Improvement in bronchial squamous metaplasia in smokers treated with folate and vitamin B_{12}. J Am Med Assoc 259:1525–1530.
21. Riotton G, Christopherson WM, Lunt R (1977): Cytology of non-gynaecological sites (International Histological Classification of Tumours, No. 17). Geneva, World Health Organization.
22. Das KC, Herbert V (1978): The lymphocyte as a marker of past nutritional status: Persistence of abnormal lymphocyte deoxyuridine (dU) suppression test and chromosomes in patients with past deficiency of folate and vitamin B12. Br J Haematol 38:219–233.
23. Haltalin KC, Nelson JP, Woodman EB, Allen AA (1970): Fatal Shigella infection induced by folic acid deficiency in young guinea pigs. J Infect Dis 121:275–287.

Vitamins and Cancer Prevention, pages 51–59
© *1991 Wiley-Liss, Inc.*

5 | Folate, Vitamin B$_{12}$, and Methylation Interactions in Tumor Formation

Lionel A. Poirier, Ph.D.

INTRODUCTION

Previous studies from our laboratory demonstrated that the chronic administration of the hepatocarcinogen diethylnitrosamine (DEN) to rats resulted in a folic acid deficiency [1]. This deficiency could be reversed by the simultaneous feeding of high dietary levels of methionine and of choline, the chief sources of preformed methyl donors, but not by the similar feeding of vitamin B$_{12}$ or of folic acid, the vitamins chiefly responsible for the de novo biosynthesis of methyl groups (Table I). These studies on the folic acid deficiency in carcinogenesis began with the observation that the chronic administration of DEN to rats, which were subsequently given a loading dose of histidine, resulted in an elevated excretion of the histidine metabolite, formiminoglutamic acid (FIGLU) [1]. Formiminoglutamic acid excretion generally reflects an insufficiency of active folate cofactors, but it can result indirectly from deficiencies of the other lipotropic agents, methionine, choline, and vitamin B$_{12}$. While high dietary levels of methionine and/or

Division of Comparative Toxicology, National Center for Toxicological Research, Jefferson, Arkansas 72079

TABLE I. The Effect of 3-Weeks' Feeding of DEN (100 ppm in Drinking Water) on the Hepatic Levels of Methionine Intermediates and Enzymes

Substance	Unit	Hepatic level[a]		DEN + methionine[b]	Reference
		Control	DEN		
SAM	μg/gm	26.6 ± 1.9	19.4 ± 0.8[c]	27.4 ± 3.3	2
Pteroyl polyglutamates	μg/gm	18.7 ± 1.1	11.8 ± 2.2[c]	22.4 ± 2.9	1
Methylcobalamin	% of total	0.72 ± 0.18	0.98 ± 0.21		3
Methionine synthase	μmol/μg protein/hr	0.14 ± 0.01	0.11 ± 0.00[c]		2
Methylenetetra-hydrofolate reductase	μmol/μg protein/hr	0.31 ± 0.02	0.35 ± 0.02		2

[a]Mean ± SEM (5–6 animals per group).
[b]1.5% in the diet.
[c]Significantly different from control.

choline suppressed the elevated levels of FIGLU excretion in DEN-treated rats, similar treatment with high dietary levels of folic acid or vitamin B_{12} had no such effect. Thus, the two dietary sources of preformed methyl donors, methionine and choline, inhibited at least one of the metabolic abnormalities produced by DEN. We then undertook a series of studies to determine the mechanism by which the dietary methyl donors exerted their effects on the elevated excretion of FIGLU in DEN-treated rats [1–3]. These results are illustrated in Table I. A number of hepatic parameters were determined to detect which were directly responsible for the reversal of the elevated FIGLU excretions. Of all biochemical intermediates examined, two were associated with the methionine-sparing effects on FIGLU excretion: pteroylpolyglutamates and S-adenosylmethionine (SAM) (Table I). Thus, the reduced hepatic levels of SAM with its consequent development of a hepatic folate insufficiency appeared to be the mechanism by which DEN produced the elevated levels of urinary FIGLU [4].

METHIONINE AND CHOLINE

The role of methionine and choline in carcinogenesis was therefore examined by the use of amino acid defined diets. These diets, in which levels of each of the amino acids are completely controlled, permitted the regulation of the hepatic SAM content by controlling the dietary levels of methionine, choline, vitamin B_{12}, and folic acid. For this purpose, we developed a standard protocol by which male weaning F-344 rats were given a single initiating dose of 20 mg/kg of DEN and subsequently placed on amino acid

TABLE II. Liver Tumor Formation in Male F-344 Rats Receiving a Single Initiating Dose of Diethylnitrosamine (DEN) and Subsequently Fed an Amino Acid Defined, Methyl-Deficient Diet[a,b]

Diet number	Methionine	Choline	% of animals dying with liver tumors[c] during the 78 weeks following DEN initiation at			
			0	20	70	200
				(mg/kg)		
1	+	+	0	0	48	54
2	−	−	54	96	93	93
3	−	+		14	65	85
4	+	−		8	46	63

[a]From [5].
[b]Male weanling rats (30 per group) were fed diet No. 1 for 1 week, injected with DEN, fed diet No. 1 for an additional week, and then placed on the promoting diet.
[c]Hepatocellular carcinomas.

defined diets whose contents of methionine, choline, folic acid, and vitamin B_{12} were completely controlled. In this study four diets were used:

Diet 1.   An adequate diet that contained both methionine and choline.
Diet 2.   A deficient diet lacking both methionine and choline.
Diet 3.   A diet lacking methionine only.
Diet 4.   A diet lacking choline only.

In Diets 2 and 3, methionine was replaced with equimolar homocystine. These diets were fed for 18 months after which all survivors were sacrificed [5]. This series of investigations demonstrated that dietary methyl insufficiency exerts both complete hepatocarcinogenic and liver tumor promoting activity in rats (Table II). The hepatocarcinogenicity of choline-deficient diets had previously been described [6], but had later been attributed to aflatoxin contamination (see review by Newberne [7]). Similar findings on the hepatocarcinogenic activity of dietary methyl insufficiency have been made by other groups [8,9] in rats as well as in mice [7,10]. The cocarcinogenic and liver tumor promoting activities of dietary methyl deprivation have also been previously described [11,12]. As indicated in Table III, the chronic feeding of these methyl-deficient, amino acid defined diets to rats led to decreased hepatic levels of SAM, increased levels of the methylase inhibitor *S*-adenosylhomocysteine (SAH), and a concomitant decrease in the SAM/SAH ratios [13]. The low hepatic ratio of SAM/SAH in rats fed methyl-deficient diets produces a hypomethylating environment in vivo, which is accompanied by decreased hepatic 5-methyldeoxycytidine (5-MC)

TABLE III. Effect of 5-Week Administration of Methyl-Deficient, Amino Acid Defined Diets on Hepatic Levels of SAM and SAH in Male Rats[a]

Diet	Methionine	Choline	Dietary methyl level (mmol/kg)	SAM (μg/g)	SAH (μg/g)	SAM/SAH
1	+	+	45.7	47 ± 1[b]	8 ± 1	6.2 ± 0.8
2	−	−	0	23 ± 1	14 ± 2	1.6 ± 0.2
3	−	+	14.3	22 ± 1	13 ± 1	1.7 ± 0.1
4	+	−	31.4	27 ± 1	8 ± 1	3.4 ± 0.3
5[c]	−	−	0	14 ± 1	17 ± 2	0.8 ± 0.1

[a]From [13].
[b]Results are expressed as means ± SEM (5–6 animals per group).
[c]This diet was the same as diet No. 2 except that folic acid and vitamin B_{12} were also excluded.

content [14]. Thus, a good correspondence can be seen between the bioavailability of methyl groups in vivo and the occurrence of liver cancer.

On the basis of these observations, one might predict that high dietary levels of methionine and choline would inhibit the hepatocarcinogenic or liver tumor promoting activities of more classical hepatocarcinogens. This indeed appears to be the case. For example, as shown in Table IV, high dietary levels of methionine and choline inhibit the formation of liver carcinomas in male C3H mice fed 0.05% phenobarbital (PhB) for 1 year [15]. A partial listing of hepatocarcinogens or liver tumor promoters whose activities are inhibited by the chronic administration of methionine, is shown in Table V.

VITAMIN B_{12} AND FOLIC ACID

In view of the enhancing effects that physiological methyl insufficiency exerts in hepatocarcinogenesis, it might perhaps be predicted that deficiencies of either vitamin B_{12} or of folic acid would similarly result in the enhancement of carcinogenesis. In fact, the superimposition of a folic acid and vitamin B_{12} deficiency in animals already deficient in methionine and choline leads to further decreases in hepatic SAM, increases in SAH, and decreased ratios of SAM/SAH (Table III) [13]. Other studies found that hepatic SAM content can be diminished by the single deficiency of vitamin B_{12} [22] or by folic acid deficiency in choline-deficient rats [23]. Thus, as expected, both vitamin B_{12} and folic acid modulate the bioavailability of SAM. Paradoxically, however, deficiencies of vitamin B_{12} have customarily been associated with the inhibition of carcinogenesis, rather than with its enhancement [24–26]. For example, as illustrated in Table VI, vitamin B_{12} supplementation enhances the hepatocarcinogenic activity of dimethylami-

TABLE IV. Effect of Dietary Methionine and Choline on Liver Carcinoma Formation in Male C3H Mice Fed 0.05% PhB for 1 Year[a]

Group	Dietary methyl content (mmol/kg)	% of rats with liver carcinoma	
		Control	PhB
Chow	47.8	0	79
Choline	119.4	3	74
Methionine	148.3	7	60
Methionine + choline	219.9	7	31

[a]Reference [15].

TABLE V. Hepatocarcinogens and Promoters Whose Activity Is Inhibited by the Chronic Administration of Methionine

Compound or diet	Species	Source
Dimethylaminoazobenzene	Rat	16, 17
2-Acetylaminofluorene	Rat	18, 12,[a] 19
DEN	Rat	12
Ethionine	Rat	20, 21
Phenobarbital	Mouse	15
Methyl deficiency	Rat	5
	Mouse	7, 10

[a]Methionine supplementation was combined with folate.

TABLE VI. The Effect of Vitamin B_{12} Supplementation on the Hepatocarcinogenic Activity of DEN-Fed Rats

Experiment number	Dietary supplement	Incidence of liver cancer
1[a]	None	1/6
	Vitamin B_{12}	7/9
	Methionine	1/9
	Vitamin B_{12} + methionine	3/9
2[b]	None	6/16
	Vitamin B_{12}	14/18

[a]From [27].
[b]From [28].

noazobenzene in rats [27,28]. We therefore examined the effects of vitamin B_{12} and folic acid on the tumor-promoting activities of methyl deprivation. We found that vitamin B_{12} deficiency inhibited the tumor-promoting activity of the methyl-deficient diets (Table VII) [29]. Decreasing the vitamin B_{12} content in the diet from 50 to 0.5 μg/kg lowered the tumor incidence from 90 to 35% in animals receiving a single initiating dose of DEN and subsequently fed the methionine- and choline-deficient diets customarily used in this laboratory. Folate deficiency exhibited a similar, but less marked, effect

TABLE VII. The Effect of Vitamin B$_{12}$ Deficiency on Liver Tumor Formation in Male Weanling F-344 Rats Given a Single Initiating Dose of DEN (20 mg/kg) and Subsequently Fed Methionine- and Choline-Deficient Diets for 18 Months[a]

Group number	Vitamin B$_{12}$ in diet (μg/kg)	Percent survival at 40 weeks	Weight gain at 10 weeks	Liver tumor incidence[b] (%)
1	50	95	68	90
2	15	96	61	75
3	5	12	49	36
4	1.5	0	32	29
5	0.5	0	30	35

[a]From [29].
[b]Includes both benign and malignant tumors.

TABLE VIII. The Effect of Folic Acid Deficiency on Liver Carcinoma Formation in Methionine- and Choline-Deficient Rats Receiving a Single Initiating Dose of DEN[a,b]

Group	Folate (mg/kg)	Weight gain at 10 weeks (gm)	Cumulative proportion with carcinomas at month			
			6	12	18	Final
1	5.0	68	0/0	1/2	3/5	18/20
2	1.5	77	0/0	1/2	5/6	16/23
3	0.5	78	0/0	1/1	9/12	18/24
4	0.15	78	0/0	0/0	4/5	11/22[c]
5	0.05	83	0/0	1/2	5/7	13/23[c]

[a]From [29].
[b]The diets contained the standard level of vitamin B$_{12}$ (50 μg/kg).
[c]Significantly different from Group 1 controls ($P < 0.02$).

with these diets (Table VIII) [29]. In the latter study, decreasing the folate content from 5 to 0.05–0.15 mg/kg lowered the final incidence of carcinomas from 90 to approximately 55% (Table VIII). Interestingly, however, folate deficiency increased the development of cholangiolar and other non-hepatocellular tumors in the livers of methionine- and choline-deficient rats (Table IX) [29]. In addition, vitamin B$_{12}$ deficiency had two other significant effects on carcinogenesis in rats initiated with DEN and subsequently fed the methionine- and choline-deficient diets. First, vitamin B$_{12}$ deficiency lowered the proportion of hepatocellular carcinomas that developed metastases in the methionine- and choline-deficient rats. Thus, while 36% (28/77) of the vitamin B$_{12}$-adequate rats fed the methyl-deficient diets and bearing hepatocellular carcinomas developed metastases, only 7% (1/15) of the corresponding vitamin B$_{12}$-deficient animals did so [29]. Also, vitamin B$_{12}$ deficiency led to the formation of forestomach papillomas in the methyl-deficient rats (Table X). While none of the rats given a single initiating dose

TABLE IX. The Effect of Vitamin B$_{12}$ and Folic Acid Deficiencies on the Development of Cholangiolar and Other Nonhepatocellular Tumors in the Livers of Methionine- and Choline-Deficient Rats Given a Single Initiating Dose of DEN

Combined groups	Proportion of animals developing nonhepatocellular liver tumors at			
	6–12 months	12–18 months	terminal sacrifice	total
B$_{12}$ and folate adequate	0/2	0/8	0/11	0/21
Folate deficient	0/5	7/32	16/57[a]	23/94[b]
B$_{12}$ deficient	2/63	2/15	1/3[a]	5/81
B$_{12}$ and folate deficient	0/27	0/0	0/0	0/27

[a]Significantly different from corresponding B$_{12}$- and folate-adequate group ($0.01 < p < 0.05$).
[b]Significantly different from corresponding B$_{12}$- and folate-adequate group ($p < 0.01$).

TABLE X. The Effects of Vitamin B$_{12}$ on the Incidence of Forestomach Squamous Papillomas in DEN-Initiated Rats Subsequently Fed a Methionine- and Choline-Deficient Diet[a]

Combined groups	Incidence	Percent
Vitamin B$_{12}$ adequate	0/113	0
Vitamin B$_{12}$ deficient	11/131*	8.4

[a]From [29].
*$p < 0.005$.

of DEN and subsequently fed a methionine-and choline-deficient diet that was also adequate in vitamin B$_{12}$ developed forestomach squamous papillomas (0/113), 8.4% (11/131) of the rats fed the corresponding vitamin B$_{12}$-deficient diet did develop such tumors [29]. No forestomach papillomas were seen in any animals not receiving an initiating dose of DEN.

Finally, just as deficiencies of vitamin B$_{12}$ and/or folate alter the bioavailability of SAM, single and combined deficiencies of methionine and choline alter the distribution of cobalamin cofactors in several tissues [30]. For example, as illustrated in Table XI, deficiencies of methionine, choline, and vitamin B$_{12}$ alter differently the hepatic contents of total cobalamins and of methylcobalamins (MeCbl) (Table XI). Thus, methionine deficiency alone increased the proportion of MeCbl in the livers of rats compared to the corresponding levels in methionine-adequate animals. Also, choline deficiency alone lowered the total cobalamin content in liver as much as did a vitamin B$_{12}$ deficiency for the same 2 weeks' feeding period.

SUMMARY

In summary, the present investigations show: (1) that dietary methyl deprivation exerts significant carcinogenic and tumor-promoting activities in the livers or rodents; (2) that such activities are modulated by the superimposi-

TABLE XI. The Effect of 2-Weeks' Feeding of Methyl-Deficient, Amino Acid Defined Diets on the Hepatic Contents of Methylcobalamin (MeCbl) in Male Weaning Rats[a]

Diet number	Constitutent added			Cobalamins[b]		
	Methionine	Choline	B_{12}	Total (pg/mg)	MeCbl (pg/mg)	% MeCbl
1	+	+	+	67 ± 13	1.6 ± 0.5	2.4 ± 0.7
2	+	+	−	19 ± 1	0.5 ± 0.2	3.0 ± 1.4
3	−	+	+	49 ± 9	4.4 ± 1.5	8.5 ± 1.6
4	−	+	−	24 ± 4	0.8 ± 0.3	3.0 ± 1.0
5	−	−	−	25 ± 2	0.2 ± 0.1	0.8 ± 0.4
6	−	−	−	43 ± 6	0.2 ± 0.1	0.4 ± 0.3
7	+	−	+	20 ± 3	0.1 ± 0.1	0.6 ± 0.3
8	+	−	−	7 ± 1	0 ± 0	0 ± 0

[a]From [30].
[b]Mean ± SEM of 5 rats per group.

tion of dietary deficiencies of vitamin B_{12} and folic acid; and (3) that the de novo and preformed sources of methyl donors exert strong effects on the metabolism of each other in vivo.

REFERENCES

1. Poirier LA, Whitehead VM (1973): Folate deficiency and elevated formiminoglutamate excretion during chronic diethylnitrosamine administration to rats. Cancer Res 33:383–388.
2. Buehring YSS, Poirier LA, Stokstad ELR (1976): Folate deficiency in the livers of diethylnitrosamine-treated rats. Cancer Res 36:2775–2779.
3. Linnell JC, Quadros EV, Matthews DM, Morris HP, and Poirier LA (1977): Altered cobalamin distribution in rat hepatomas and in the livers of rats treated with diethylnitrosamine. Cancer Res 37:2975–2978.
4. Kutzbach CA, Stokstad ELR (1967): Feedback inhibition of methylenetetrahydrofolate reductase in rat liver by S-adenosylmethionine. Biochim Biophys Acta 139:217–220.
5. Mikol YB, Hoover KL, Creasia D, Poirier LA (1983): Hepatocarcinogenesis in rats fed methyl-deficient, amino acid-defined diets. Carcinogenesis 4:1619–1629.
6. Copeland DH, Salmon WD (1946): The occurrence of neoplasms in the liver, lungs, and other tissues of rats as a result of prolonged choline deficiency. Am J Pathol 22:1059–1079.
7. Newberne PM (1986): Lipotropic factors and oncogenesis. In Poirier LA, Pariza MW, Newberne PM (eds): "Essential Nutrients in Carcinogenesis," New York: Plenum, pp 223–251.
8. Ghoshal AK, Farber E (1984): The induction of liver cancer by dietary deficiency of choline and methionine without added carcinogens. Carcinogenesis 5:1367–1370.
9. Yokoyama S, Sells MA, Reddy QV, Lombardi B (1985): Hepatocarcinogenic and promoting action of a choline-devoid diet in the rat. Cancer Res 45:2834–2842.
10. Poirier LA, Hoover K (1986): Liver tumor formation in male B6C3F1 mice fed methyl-deficient, amino acid-defined diets with and without diethylnitrosamine initiations. Proc Am Assoc Cancer Res 27:129 (abstract).

11. Shinozuka H, Katyal SL, Perera MIR (1986): Fats, lipotropes, hypolipidemic agents, and liver cancer. In Clement IP, Birt DR, Rogers AE, Mettlin C (eds): "Dietary Fat and Cancer," New York: Liss, pp 461–486.

12. Rogers AE, Newberne PM (1980): Lipotrope deficiency in experimental carcinogenesis. Nutr Cancer 2:104.

13. Shivapurkar N, Poirier LA (1983): Tissues levels of S-adenosylmethionine in rats fed methyl-deficient, amino acid-defined diets for one to five weeks. Carcinogenesis 4:1051–1057.

14. Wilson MJ, Shivapurkar N, Poirier LA (1984): Hypomethylation of hepatic nuclear DNA in rats fed with a carcinogenic methyl-deficient diet. Biochem J 218:987–990.

15. Poirier LA, Mikol YB, Hoover K, Creasia D (1984): The inhibition by methionine and choline of liver carcinoma formation in male C3H mice fed phenobarbital. Proc Am Assoc Cancer Res 25:132 (abstract).

16. Miller JA, Miller EC (1953): The carcinogenic aminoazo dyes. Adv Cancer Res 1:339–396.

17. Terayama H (1967): Aminoazo carcinogenesis—methods and biochemical problems. In Busch H (ed): "Methods in Cancer Research," New York: Academic, pp 399–449.

18. Miller EC, Miller JA (1972): Approaches to the mechanisms and control of chemical carcinogenesis. In "Environment and Cancer," University of Texas at Houston and M.D. Anderson Hospital and Tumor Institute, Baltimore: Williams & Wilkins, pp 5–39.

19. Brada Z, Altman NH, Hill M, Bulba S (1984): Effect of methionine (M) on progression of tumors induced by *N-2-fluorenylacetamide* (FAA). Fed Proc 43:591 (abstract).

20. Farber E (1963): Ethionine carcinogenesis. Adv Cancer Res 7:383–474.

21. Brada Z, Altman NH, Hill M, Bulba S (1982): The effect of methionine on the progression of hepatocellular carcinoma induced by ethionine. Res Commun Chem Pathol Pharmacol 38:157–160.

22. Mikol YB, Poirier LA (1981): An inverse correlation between hepatic ornithine decarboxylase and S-adenosylmethionine in rats. Cancer Res 13:195–201.

23. Henning SM, McKee RW, Swendseid ME (1989): Hepatic content of S-adenosylmethionine, S-adenosylhomocysteine, and glutathione in rats receiving treatments modulating methyl donor availability. J Nutr 119:1478–1482.

24. Myasishcheva NV (1974): Characteristics of the metabolism of vitamin B_{12} compounds (cobalamins) during leukoses. In Raushenbakh MO (ed), "Role of Endogenous Factors in the Development of Leukoses," Meditsina, Moscow, pp 1–69.

25. Herbert V (1986): The role of vitamin B_{12} and folate in carcinogenesis. In Poirier LA, Pariza MW, Newberne PM (eds): "Essential Nutrients in Carcinogenesis," New York: Plenum, pp 293–311.

26. Eto I, Krumdieck CL (1986): Role of vitamin B_{12} and folate deficiencies in carcinogenesis. In Poirier LA, Pariza MW, Newberne PM (eds): "Essential Nutrients in Carcinogenesis," New York: Plenum, pp 313–330.

27. Day PL, Payne LD, Dinning JS (1950): Procarcinogenic effect of vitamin B_{12} on *p*-dimethylaminoazobenzene-fed rats. Proc Soc Exptl Biol Med 74:854–857.

28. Miller EC, Plescia AM, Miller JA, Heidelberger CH (1952): Metabolism of methylated aminoazo dyes. I. The demethylation of 3′-methyl-4-dimethyl-C^{14}-aminobenzene *in vivo*. J Biol Chem 196:863–874.

29. Poirier LA, Hoover KL, Ward JM (1987): Effects of vitamin B_{12} and folate on hepatocarcinogenesis in choline/methionine-deficient (CMD) rats. Fed Proc 46:750 (abstract).

30. Linnell JC, Wilson MJ, Mikol YB, Poirier LA (1983): Tissue distribution of methylcobalamin in rats fed amino acid-defined, methyl-deficient diets. J Nutr 113:124–130.

Vitamins and Cancer Prevention, pages 61–90
© *1991 Wiley-Liss, Inc.*

6 | Vitamins E and C in Neoplastic Development

Mary P. Carpenter, Ph.D.

Department of Molecular Toxicology, Oklahoma Medical Research Foundation, and Department of Biochemistry and Molecular Biology, University of Oklahoma Health Sciences Center, Oklahoma City, Oklahoma 73104

PROPERTIES AND BIOLOGICAL EFFECTS OF
VITAMINS E AND C

Introduction

The hypothesis that free radicals have a role in carcinogenesis has stimulated interest in the potential roles of vitamins E and C as potential inhibitors of tumorigenesis. The antioxidant activity of vitamins E and C are well documented. A variety of observations suggest that free radicals may be implicated in the etiology of cancer. Carcinogenesis is enhanced under conditions in which free radicals are produced; tumor promoters stimulate the generation of free radicals. Free radicals could have early roles in cancer; oxidative mechanisms have an important role in activating certain carcinogens. Antioxidants and free radical scavengers inhibit tumorigenesis. Several cellular targets, cellular proteins and/or enzymes, membrane lipids, and DNA, are potentially vulnerable to free radical attack. Neither the nature of the free radicals implicated, nor the site of their action, nor the stage of tumorigenesis affected, have been unequivocally clarified.

Support for oxygen-centered free radical mediated events includes the results of a variety of studies indicating that oxygen enhances radiation-induced carcinogenesis and mutation [1]. The activities of peroxidases, lipoxygenases, prostaglandin synthase, and lipid peroxidation of membrane polyenoic fatty acids generate peroxides and hydroperoxides. Free radicals generated from these compounds are believed to be active molecules in tumor promotion.

Endogenous systems that afford protection from free radical damage include glutathione generation as well as the activities of catalase, superoxide dismutases, and glutathione peroxidases. Free radicals generated during the course of lipid peroxidation of cellular membranes have been postulated to be important mediators in carcinogenesis. This is supported by reports showing that vitamin E as well as many synthetic antioxidants inhibit tumor formation in a number of models of chemically induced neoplasia. Whether the protective effect(s) occur at the initiation or promotion phase of carcinogenesis, or both, is not clear.

Ascorbate is a good reducing agent, which is known to affect many cellular biochemical processes including collagen synthesis, neuropeptide synthesis and function, and to influence immune function. Vitamin E is an integral component of cellular membranes. The antioxidant function of vitamin E, the reducing action of ascorbate, and potential in vivo synergism between vitamins E and C may play a role in modulating neoplasia.

The objective of this chapter is to examine the current status of the role(s) of vitamins E and C in cancer. Evidence considered includes epidemiological studies of correlations between vitamin E and C status and cancer risk in humans, as well as the results of studies utilizing a number of animal cancer models, with emphasis on work published during the past few years.

Properties of Vitamin E

Structure and chemistry. The term vitamin E refers to tocopherols, fat soluble vitamins, consisting of a chroman ring and a 16 carbon phytyl side chain, which confers upon the molecule its hydrophobic properties. Methyl substitutions and the presence of an hydroxyl group on the ring are important for function. For example, the most biologically active form of vitamin E, α-tocopherol [2,5,7,8-tetramethyl-2(4′,8′,12′-trimethyltridecyl)-6-chromanol], has methyl groups on the 5,7, and 8 carbon atoms and an hydroxyl group at carbon atom 6.

Role in membranes and cells. The role of vitamin E in the biology of cells has not been clarified. Symptoms of vitamin E deficiency tend to be species specific and include the skeletomuscular, reproductive, neural, and vascular systems. A deficiency syndrome that transcends a broad spectrum of species is disrupted gametogenesis. Abnormal gamete differentiation occurs in vitamin E deficiency in insects, birds, fishes, and a variety of mammals.

As an integral component of membranes, vitamin E has effects on the physicochemical and physiological properties of membranes. The localization of vitamin E within the structure of the membrane is critical to its role as a membrane antioxidant and stabilizer. Free radical scavenging by vitamin E is believed to prevent oxidant injury to membrane polyunsaturated fatty acids, to proteins rich in thiols, and to the cellular cytoskeleton. The molecule is amphipathic; the chromanol head group is oriented in the membrane toward the hydrophilic face of the bilayer and the phytyl side chain intercalates between the unsaturated fatty acid side chains of the hydrophobic interior of the bilayer [2–6]. The presence of α-tocopherol in the bilayer affects membrane fluidity [7–9]. In addition to affecting the physical properties and organization of the membrane, vitamin E, as the exclusive antioxidant present in membranes, is believed to provide the cell with a defense mechanism against oxidative stress by, for example, inhibiting the peroxidation of membrane polyenoic fatty acids. Compared to the amounts of polyenoic fatty acids, however, the amount of vitamin E in a membrane is very small.

Vitamin E is regenerated in the presence of ascorbic acid [10–12]. Tappel [2] was one of the first to suggest that the tocopheroxyl free radical form of vitamin E might be regenerated. Early evidence to support this concept were the in vitro studies of Packer et al. [13] who were able to demonstrate that α-tocopherol was regenerated in the presence of ascorbate, and that in this cycle, a dehydroascorbate radical is formed.

Properties of Vitamin C

Structure and chemistry. Vitamin C (L,3-ketothreohexuronic acid lactone) is commonly referred to as ascorbic acid (L-ascorbic acid). Ascorbic acid is a one-electron carrier and acts as a reductant as it is easily oxidized to dehydroascorbic acid. The bioavailability of inorganic iron is enhanced by vitamin C, which can reduce ferric iron (Fe^{3+}) to the more readily absorbed ferrous (Fe^{2+}) ion. In the presence of oxygen and iron ascorbate catalyzes the hydroxylation of a variety of compounds.

Ascorbic acid is synthesized by most animals. Notable exceptions are the human, other primates and the guinea pig which do not have an active L-gulonolactone oxidase, and thus require dietary vitamin C.

Role in cells. In humans, the adrenal gland contains the highest concentration of ascorbate (400–500 mg/100 g of fresh tissue). Ascorbate is required for development of a normal skeleton. Ascorbic acid deficiency and malnutrition result in osteoporosis. Vitamin C was originally believed to have a metabolic role related to its reversible oxidation and reduction. However, a specific oxidation system in which ascorbic acid serves as a specific coenzyme has not been documented. Morre et al. [14], described an NADH ferricyanide reductase that utilizes an ascorbate free radical, which is postulated to function as an electron receptor for this NADH-free radical reductase. Free radical forms of ascorbate are the semidehydro and monodehydro, which are formed from dehydroascorbate. Vitamin C in its role in supporting hydroxylation facilitates removal of iron from ferritin. Ascorbate is also involved in the hydroxylation of proline. As a reducing agent, ascorbic acid maintains prolyl hydroxylase in an active form by keeping the iron atom in the reduced form. Most of the symptoms of scurvy (vitamin C deficiency) reflect problems with the formation of collagen and chondroitin sulfate. Ascorbate is believed to be an inducer of the collagen pathway [15]. Recent studies suggest that vitamin C, as a cofactor for monooxygenase, is an essential cofactor for peptide neurotransmitter synthesis [16].

VITAMIN E AND CANCER—HUMAN SUBJECTS

Information on vitamin E and cancer in humans has only recently become available. The results of epidemiological studies of fairly large human populations suggest that there may be an inverse correlation between increased risk for certain types of cancer and serum concentrations of tocopherol. The epidemiological studies are complicated by methodological problems, which include the statistical analytical techniques used as well as difficulties with procedures for optimal procurement, storage, and analysis of the biological samples collected.

Epidemiological Studies

Cancer in general. Salonen et al. [17] in a prospective study found an inverse relationship between α-tocopherol and the overall risk of cancer and cancer death, especially in nonsmoking men. However, in regard to cancer in general, several other epidemiological studies indicate no association of serum vitamin E levels and cancer risk at any of the sites examined [18–20]. In a prospective study of 20,000 British men, Wald et al. [21] observed no differences between serum α-tocopherol values of the subjects who developed cancer and those of appropriately matched, healthy controls. Although sera of subjects developing cancer within a year of the date blood was collected had significantly lower levels, these low α-tocopherol values were considered not to be predictive, but to reflect the disease state.

Breast cancer. The correlations between serum concentrations of vitamin E and breast cancer risk are ambiguous. Wald et al. [22] observed a significant association of low serum tocopherol levels with an increased risk for mammary neoplasia, but later [23] suggested their 1984 results may have been artifactual and that the low values they had previously reported might have been consequences of losses of vitamin E during storage and freeze–thawing of samples. Russel et al. [24] studied a population similar to that of Wald, and found no differences in tocopherol levels in those subjects with breast cancer as compared to controls. A similar lack of correlation was made in a study of ovarian cancer [25]. In apparent contrast to the above studies, in which there appear not to be differences as compared to controls, in a hospital based case control study of breast cancer patients in Milan, Italy and Montpellier, France, the plasma tocopherol values of the cancer patients were higher than the controls and there was a 4.2 times increased risk in the highest quadrille [26]. Langeman et al. [27] found no differences in the tocopherol content of samples of neoplastic and nonneoplastic breast tissue from the same patients.

Gastrointestinal and lung cancer. A study, planned in 1960 as a survey of cardiovascular disease in 6300 healthy volunteers working for a pharmaceutical firm, the Basel study [18], has also turned out to be a prospective study of vitamins E and C and cancer death. Plasma vitamins (vitamins E and C, and β-carotene) were measured in 1971–1973. A mortality follow-up carried out in 1980 showed that 4% of the total deaths (10%) were cancer-related [28, 29]. In a 7-year follow-up, Gey et al. [29] observed a lower vitamin E concentration in samples of subjects whose deaths were related to gastrointestinal, as well as all other cancers. The findings of Knekt et al. [30], in a longitudinal study of a large population (36,000 Finnish subjects) with a 6–10-year follow-up, documented that the serum vitamin E of subjects who developed gastrointestinal cancer was low as compared to matched controls and reflected a 2.2-fold increase in risk for upper gastrointestinal cancer. The correlation was stronger for men than women. There was no association with colon cancer, which contrasts with an inverse relationship between plasma α-tocopherol and colon cancer reported by Stähelin et al. [18]. In a similar study among 21,000 Finnish men with a follow-up of 6–10 years, high serum tocopherol was associated with a reduced risk for overall cancer [31]. When the risks for the two highest and two lowest quadrilles were adjusted for other factors, such as smoking and blood cholesterol level, the data supported a decreased risk for those cancers unrelated to smoking— stomach, pancreas, and urinary bladder. In a longitudinal study of 15,000 Finnish women, there was an inverse relationship between low serum vitamin E values and the development of hormone-related cancers during an 8-year follow-up, with a 1.6-fold increase in risk between the two highest and the two lowest quadrilles [32].

Current status. There are no reports of cancer clinical trials using vitamin E. A recent report comparing the effects of vitamin E and selenium during cytotoxic chemotherapy of gynecological cancer does not document a protective role [33]. The various epidemiological studies on vitamin E and cancer, neither utilize identical protocols nor assess the same general populations. However, these studies do provide some evidence to support a role for vitamin E in cancer of specific tissues, especially the upper gastrointestinal tract. A recent report [34] suggests that a 12-year follow-up of the Basel study no longer supports a statistically significant lower serum vitamin E concentration in patients when separated into gastrointestinal cancer or in all cancer as had been observed in the 7-year follow-up study [29]. However, in agreement with others [32,35,36] the tendency remained for lung cancer to be associated with low serum values for vitamin E. Menkes et al. [35] and Miyamoto et al. [37] found that serum vitamin E levels were significantly lower in lung cancer cases. Stähelin et al. [34] conclude that low serum vitamin E levels are associated with an overall increased risk for cancer, but that the association is not very strong. Thus, epidemiological evidence for a protective role for vitamin E in cancer prevention remains conflictory.

VITAMIN C AND CANCER—HUMAN SUBJECTS

Introduction

Differences in the incidence of several types of cancer, apparently reflecting a high dietary intake of citrus fruit, rich sources of ascorbic acid, suggested that vitamin C might have a protective effect in cancer. Studies on the potential role of vitamin C in human cancer are limited; very few epidemiological analyses or clinical trials have been carried out. Most of the epidemiological reports assess the ascorbate status of the subjects using indirect estimations of the vitamin C content of the foods consumed by subjects using the dietary recall procedure. A protective effect of dietary ascorbate has been reported for cancer at various sites—esophageal, gastrointestinal, lung, colorectal, and oral.

Epidemiological Studies

Esophageal cancer. Based on the consumption of foods, Hormozdiari et al. [38] and Mettlin et al. [39] concluded that there was an inverse relationship between a low dietary intake of ascorbate and esophageal cancer. Cook-Mozaffari et al. [40] reached a similar conclusion in a case-control study. A high esophageal cancer incidence in an area of northern China has been attributed to low levels of vitamin C [41].

Gastrointestinal cancer. An early report [42] based on food consumption data, indicated a protective role of ascorbic acid in gastrointestinal cancer. A more recent comprehensive study in which vitamin C was assessed in serum samples supports this association. One of the few epidemiological studies on vitamin C and cancer, not based on food consumption, is the Basel study [28,29]. Serum samples of about 3000 males were analyzed for amounts of vitamin C and other vitamins in 1971 with a follow-up in 1980 and correlated with cancer death. The overall mortality was about 10%, with 4% of the deaths cancer related. Decreased amounts of serum ascorbate were associated with a statistically significant higher mortality of subjects with gastrointestinal cancer, but not with lung cancer or cancer at other sites.

Colorectal cancer. In contrast to the protective role of vitamin C in gastrointestinal cancer, neither the studies of Graham et al. [43] nor Jain et al. [44] found a correlation between dietary ascorbate and colorectal cancer.

Lung cancer. A recent report ascribes a protective effect of vitamin C, determined from food intake using a dietary questionnaire, on lung cancer risk in Louisiana [45]. A strong, inverse association between risk of squamous and small cell carcinomas and dietary intake of vitamin C was documented. However, several other groups have found no correlation between dietary ascorbate and lung cancer [46,47].

Other sites. The incidence of oral cancer was found to correlate with a decrease in dietary vitamin C [48]. A protective effect of dietary ascorbic acid on laryngeal cancer was also observed in a case-controlled study [49].

Clinical studies. While there is some epidemiological evidence that vitamin C may lower the risk for cancer at several sites, the results of limited clinical studies do not give much support for a beneficial role of vitamin C in the treatment of cancer. Although Cameron and Pauling [50] reported that pharmacological doses of ascorbic acid elicited a prolongation of survival in subjects with advanced cases of cancer, others have not corroborated this

TABLE I. Effect of Vitamin E on Cancer in Animal Models—Various Sites

Carcinogen[a]	Animal model	Parameters tested[a]	Result	Reference
Bladder				
BBN	Rat	Antioxidants, hyperplasia	No effect of vitamin E	58
Colon				
DMH	Rat	Tumors	Decreased incidence	59
DMH	Rat	Vitamin E deficiency, tumors	No effect	60
DMH	Rat	Tumors	Decreased incidence	61
DMH	Mouse	Tumors	Increased incidence	62
Gastrointestinal				
MNNG	Rat	Tumors, BHT, vitamins C and A	Decreased incidence (E + C)	63
MNNG	Rat	Tumors, NaCL and antioxidants	No effect of vitamin E	64
BHA	Rat	BHA and antioxidants on hyperplasia	BHA + vitamin E inhibited	65
Liver				
DEN, AAF	Rat	Hyperplastic nodules, GGT	Inhibition of initiation	66
DOPN	Hamster	Hyperplastic nodules	Inhibition by vitamin E	67
Mammary				
DMBA	Rat	Dietary fat, tumors	Enhanced in vitamin E deficient	68
DMBA	Rat	Selenium, tumors	Se protection enhanced	69
DMBA	Rat	Antioxidants, tumors	No effect of vitamin E	70
DMBA	Rat	Selenium, tumors	Se protection immune system enhanced	71
MNU	Rat	Tumors	No effect of vitamin E	72

(*continued*)

TABLE I. Effect of Vitamin E on Cancer in Animal Models—Various Sites (Continued)

Carcinogen[a]	Animal model	Parameters tested[a]	Result	Reference
Oral				
DMBA	Hamster	Tumors buccal pouch	Oral protects	73
DMBA	Hamster	Tumors buccal	Topical protects	74
DMBA	Hamster	Tumor regression and TNF	Promoted tumor regression and TNF	75
DMBA	Hamster	Buccal pouch ODC activity	Vitamin E enhanced	76
Pancreas				
Azaserine	Rat	Vitamins E, C, and A on ductal lesions	Vitamin E inhibited basophilic	77
BOP	Hamster	Vitamins E, C, and A on ductal lesions	No effect of vitamin E	77
DOPN	Hamster	Pancreatic hyperplasia	Inhibition by vitamin E	67
Skin				
DMBA, TPA	Mouse	GSH, vitamin E on ODC and tumors	Inhibition of ODC and tumors by vitamin E	78
DMBA, TPA	Mouse	Complete vs two-stage	Inhibition in two-stage but not complete	79
DMBA, TPA	Mouse	Papillomas and antioxidants	No effect of vitamin E	80

[a]Abbreviations: AAF, 2-acetylaminofluorene; BHA, butylated hydroxyanisole; BHT, butylated hydroxytoluene; BOP, *n*-nitrosobis(2-oxopropy)amine; BBN, *N*-butyl-*N*-(4-hydroxybutyl) nitrosamine; DEN, diethylnitrosamine; DMBA, 7,12-dimethylbenz(*a*)anthracene; DMH, 1,2-dimethylhydrazine; DOPN, 2,2-dioxo-*N*-nitrosodipropylamine; GGT, γ-glutamyltranspeptidase; GSH, glutathione; MNNG, *N*-methyl-*N'*-nitro-*N*-nitrosoguanidine; MNU, methylnitrosourea; ODC, ornithine decarboxylase activity; PrG, propyl gallate; α-Tph, α-tocopherol; TNF, tumor necrosis factor; TPA, 12-*O*-tetradecanoyl-phorbol-13-acetate.

effect. The controlled, double-blind studies of the Mayo Clinic group [51,52] in which high doses of ascorbic acid were given to subjects with cancer at various sites (colorectal, stomach, lung, pancreatic, etc.) revealed no differences in survival time or symptoms in the vitamin C-treated group as compared to controls. McKeown-Eyssen et al. [53] in a double-blind, randomized trial found no association between vitamins E and C and the prevention of recurrence of colorectal polyps, which are presumed to be precursors of rectal cancer. On the other hand, a modest suppressive effect of vitamin C was noted on adenomas of the rectum in patients with polyposis [54].

The concentration of vitamin C in neoplastic human tissue may be elevated as compared to normal tissue. Langemann et al. [27] found an increased content of ascorbic acid in the epithelium of neoplastic human breast tissue as compared to nonneoplastic tissue. Ascorbate was also elevated in epithelial tumors of skin compared to controls [55]. After treatment with megadoses of vitamin C, the ascorbate content of the tumor did not increase very much (15%), suggesting that the tumor is not concentrating ascorbate at the expense of the surrounding tissue [56]. Cancer therapy can influence amounts of ascorbic acid in the circulation. The results of a National Cancer Institute extramural group study of patients with metastatic cancer (melanoma, hypernephroma, and colonic) indicate that immunotherapy using high doses of interleukin 2, results in very marked decreases in plasma ascorbate concentrations [57].

EFFECTS OF VITAMINS E AND C ON CANCER IN ANIMAL MODELS
Vitamin E and Cancer—Animal Models

The effect of vitamin E on chemical carcinogen-induced cancer in animal models has been tested using a number of different animal species (mouse, rat, and hamster) and a variety of carcinogens that produce neoplasia at different sites (Table I). Although the most common endpoint of the studies is tumor incidence, other parameters of carcinogenesis were monitored in some of the investigations (see Table I). There is considerable variation in the effect of vitamin E among the models and in some cases in the results from different groups using the same model. Some of these differences may reflect differences in carcinogen dosage or chronology of treatments, as well as other factors. All the species utilized as experimental models have a dietary requirement for vitamin E.

Bladder. N-Butyl-N-(4-hydroxybutyl)nitrosamine (BBN)-initiated bladder carcinogenesis in the rat has been shown to be promoted by a variety of antioxidants including sodium ascorbate [81], BHA (butylated hydroxyanisole) [82], and BHT (butylated hydroxytoluene) [81]; in contrast, α-tocopherol is not a promoter for urinary bladder lesions [58].

Colon. The effects of vitamin E on DMH (1,2-dimethylhydrazine)-initiated tumor development in the rat and in the mouse are quite different (Table I). Reports by Cook and McNamara [61] and Colacchio et al. [59], concur that dietary vitamin E decreases tumor incidence in the rat. However, another study reports no differences between tumor incidence between

DMH-treated vitamin E-deficient and vitamin E-supplemented rats [60]. In contrast to rats, in DMH-treated mice, dietary α-tocopherol enhances tumor production [62].

Gastrointestinal. The results of studies on the influence of vitamin E on gastric tumor development in MNNG (*N*-methyl-*N* '-nitrosodipropylamine)-treated rats are also contradictory (Table I). In the studies of Balansky et al. [63], rats treated with vitamin E were also supplemented with vitamin C and BHT. The design of the study does not address vitamin E alone. Nonetheless, there do not appear to be interactions between vitamins E and C. Ascorbic acid alone decreased tumor incidence, while tumor incidence in the vitamin C plus vitamin E group was similar; thus, there is no apparent synergism. In contrast to the two-stage design used by others, Balansky treated animals with antioxidant prior to carcinogen administration. Takahashi et al. [64] report no effect of 1 or 2% vitamin E during the postinitiation phase. Several other antioxidants were effective; 1% ethoxyquin increased glandular stomach tumors and 1% BHA induced and/or promoted development of tumors in the forestomach. In a study designed to test the synergism between BHA and several other antioxidants on the induction of rat forestomach lesions, Hirose et al. [65] noted that BHA plus α-tocopherol decreased the incidence of hyperplasia in the perfundic region but that α-tocopherol plus propyl gallate increased hyperplasia in the mid-region. However, these changes did not result in forestomach cancer. These results and other studies indicate that not all antioxidants that affect hyperplasia enhance carcinogenesis [83].

Liver. Early stages in hepatic carcinogenesis in both the rat and the hamster appear to be inhibited by α-tocopherol. Ura et al. [66] assessed the effects of vitamin E on hepatocarcinogenesis, from altered foci to persistent nodules, in rats initiated with DEN (diethylnitrosamine) and then subjected to partial hepatectomy or promoted with AAF (2-acetylaminofluorene). Changes that precede hepatocellular cancer were monitored, such as GGT (γ-glutamyltranspeptidase) activity and the presence of hyperplastic nodules. When given in the diet after initiation, vitamin E inhibited the induction and growth of GGT-positive foci. When given in the diet after the GGT-positive foci were already present, 1.5% vitamin E had no effect, but lower concentrations enhanced the number of foci. Vitamin E had no effect on the progression of the GGT-positive foci into preneoplastic lesions. Moore et al. [14] observed a postinitiation inhibition of liver lesions induced in the hamster by DOPN (2,2-dioxo-*N*-nitrosodipropylamine) when a diet supplemented with vitamin E was fed. Transplantable hepatic tumors have an increased content of vitamin E as compared to normal tissue [84a and b].

Mammary. Several early studies on vitamin E in mammary cancer suggested a protective effect; this is not substantiated in more recent work. Vitamin E has no effect on MNU (methylnitrosourea)-induced mammary cancer in rats [72]. Although DMBA [7,12-dimethylbenz(*a*)anthracene]-induced mammary tumorigenesis is inhibited by a number of synthetic antioxidants, the endogenous antioxidant, vitamin E, is ineffective as an inhibitor [68,70]. However, when DMBA treated rats are fed a high polyunsaturated fat diet (25% corn oil) and threshold amounts of α-tocopherol, 7.5 mg/kg, tumor incidence is enhanced (88%) as compared to the high-fat diet with adequate vitamin E, 30 mg/kg (64%) [68]. These results indicate that when dietary tocopherol is minimal, vitamin E enhances the tumor promoting effect of high polyunsaturated fat. On the other hand, vitamin E potentiates the ability of selenium to inhibit tumors induced by DMBA [69]. This effect of vitamin E is apparent only during the promotion and not the initiation phase of mammary gland DMBA carcinogenesis. The rats in this study were fed high-fat diets, 20% corn oil, ±1000 mg/kg of vitamin E, a very high dose. As a high fat diet has a promotional effect in the DMBA model, the specific effects of selenium and of vitamin E are difficult to dissect. Recent studies suggest that these agents may have an effect on immune function [71].

Oral. In the hamster buccal pouch tumorigenesis is induced by repeated topical applications of DMBA (0.5%). Administration of α-tocopherol, either orally [73] or topically [85], inhibits buccal pouch carcinogenesis significantly. When a smaller dose of DMBA (0.1%) is used, buccal pouch cancer is entirely prevented [74]. Local or topical application of beta-carotene results in tumor regression and the induction of tumor necrosis factor (TNF) in macrophages localized in the tumor area [86]. Local injections of α-tocopherol into buccal pouches of animals with established tumors also results in tumor regression and a significant increase in TNF-positive macrophages [75]. Using the same model, Calhoun et al. [76] concluded that vitamin E protects against buccal cancer by inhibiting the ODC (ornithine decarboxylase) response to DMBA. Vitamin E, alone, stimulated ODC activity; this effect was additive to that elicited by DMBA treatment.

Pancreas. Dietary vitamin E has a differential effect on the development of putative preneoplastic foci in exocrine pancreas in azaserine-treated rats as compared to BOP [*N*-nitrosobis(2-oxopropy)amine]-treated hamsters [77]. In the rat, vitamin E had an inhibitory effect on the growth of basophilic lesions. These lesions are believed to be unrelated to pancreatic carcinogenesis. In the hamster, vitamin E had no effect on either early or advanced lesions. In contrast, Moore et al. [67] treated hamsters with DOPN, which induces ductal carcinogenesis, and found that vitamin E inhibited the development of preneoplastic lesions.

Skin. Mouse skin carcinogenesis initiated with DMBA and promoted with TPA (12-*O*-tetradecanoyl-phorbol-13-acetate) is a well-studied model. There is considerable indirect evidence suggesting a role for free radicals in

TABLE II. Effect of Vitamin C on Rat Urinary Bladder Cancer

Carcinogen[a]	Animal model	Parameters tested	Results	Reference
BBN	Two-stage F-344 rat	1 vs 5%Na ascorbate	Tumor promotion by 5%	90
BBN	Two-stage F-344 rat	Na or Ca ascorbate	Promotion only by Na ascorbate	91
BBN	Two-stage F-344 rat	$NaHCO_3$, ascorbic acid	$NaHCO_3$ promotion >by ascorbate	92
BBN	Two-stage F-344 and Lewis rats	Strains, diet effects	Strain and diet affect promotion	93
ODS	Two-stage rats	Ascorbate mutant strain	Promotion by ascorbate	94
BBN, EHBN	F-344 rat two-stage and concurrent	Ascorbic acid, citric acid, Na salts	Na ascorbate promotes only in two-stage	95
MNU	F-344 Rat	BHA, BHT Na ascorbate	Promotion by Na ascorbate	82

[a]Abbreviations: BHA, butylated hydroxyanisole; BHT, butylated hydroxytoluene; BBN, butyl-N-(4-hydroxylbutyl)nitrosamine; EHBN, N-ethyl-N-(4-hydroxybutyl)nitrosamine; MNU, methylnitrosourea; ODS, osteogenic disorder Shinogi, a mutant which lacks L-gulonolactone oxidase.

the process of mouse skin tumorigenesis. Perchellet et al. [78] used this model to determine the effects of topically applied vitamin E on the ODC activity and on tumor development. Their results show that the constituent amino acids of glutathione (cysteine, glycine, and glutamate), glutathione itself, and α-tocopherol inhibit TPA-induced ODC activity, both in vivo and in vitro, and are also effective in blocking tumor promotion. The effects of vitamin E were greater in vivo than in vitro. Vitamin E does not affect the cellular GSH/GSSG ratio. In a follow-up study, the effects of combined treatments with selenium, glutathione, and vitamin E in both the complete and multistage protocols were compared [79]. Vitamin E has a maximal inhibitory effect on tumor promotion in the two-stage protocol following DMBA initiation; vitamin E plus glutathione or vitamin E plus selenium regimens both strongly inhibited promotion. However, in the complete protocol (DMBA initiation followed by repeated applications of DMBA) vitamin E in combination with either selenium or glutathione more than doubled the tumor incidence. On the other hand, in the study of Rotstein and Slaga [80], in which the two-stage model was also used, but in which papillomas, precancerous lesions, were monitored, while glutathione inhibited their formation, vitamin E was ineffective.

Cell culture. Transformation of a variety of cells in culture induced either by radiation or chemically is inhibited by vitamin E [87]. Chinese hamster

TABLE III. Effect of Vitamin C on Cancer in Animal Models—Various Sites

Carcinogen[a]	Animal model	Parameters tested[a]	Result	Reference
Colon				
DMH	Rat	Tumors, single vs multiple dose	Inhibition single dose	96
DMH	Rat	Tumors	Decreased incidence	59,97
DMH	Rat	Tumors	Increased incidence	98
Gastrointestinal				
MNNG	Rat	Vitamin C,BHT, α-Tph	Decreased incidence	63
MNNG	Rat	Tumors	No effect	99
MNU	Rat	Tumors	Decreased incidence	96
Kidney				
Estradiol or DES	Hamster	Tumors	Decreased incidence	100
Liver				
AFB	Rat	Vitamin C and other agents, tumors and survival	Decreased tumors and survival	101
Mammary				
RIII	Mice	Spontaneous tumors	Protection	102
DMBA	Mice	Tumors	No effect	103
DMBA	Rat	Inhibition of tumors by Se	Inhibited	104
	Mice	Survival time in mice injected with cancer cells	Increased	105
Melanoma				
	Mice	Ca ascorbate on survival	Increased	106
Sarcoma				
BP	Rat	Tumors	Inhibition	107
Fibrosarcoma cells	Rat	Tumors	Decreased incidence	108
3-MC	Rat	Tumors	Increased incidence	109
Transplantable tumors	Mouse	Survival time	Increased survival	110

(continued)

TABLE III. Effect of Vitamin C on Cancer in Animal Models—Various Sites (Continued)

Carcinogen[a]	Animal model	Parameters tested[a]	Result	Reference
Skin				
UV light	Mouse	Tumors	Decreased incidence	111
DMBA, TPA	Mouse	Ascorbate vs ascorbate esters on tumors and ODC	Decreased incidence	112

Abbreviations: AFB, Aflatoxin B_1; AO, antioxidant; BHA, butylated hydroxyanisole; BHT, hydroxytoluene; BOP, N-nitrosobis(2-oxypropyl)amine; BP, benzo(a)pyrene; DES, diethylstilbesterol; DMBA, 7,12-dimethylbenz(a)anthracene; DMH, 1,2-dimethyhydrazine; 3-MC, 3-methylcholanthrene; MNNG, N-methyl-N'-nitro-N-nitrosoguanidine; MNU, methylnitrosourea; ODC, ornithine decarboxylase activity; TPA, 12-O-tetradecanoyl-phorbol-13-acetate; α-Tph, α-tocopherol.

ovary cells are protected from sister chromatid exchange formation under conditions of oxygen radical-induced toxicity when vitamin E is present in the medium [88]. Vitamin E enhances cell proliferation and colony formation in an epidermoid carcinoma cell line derived from DMBA-induced tumors of buccal pouch, but inhibits at high concentrations [89].

Vitamin C and Cancer—Animal Models

The effect of vitamin C on cancer has been investigated using various strains of rats, mice, and hamsters and a number of different carcinogens. Other variables in the studies have included carcinogen dose, time of administration, and the frequency and route of treatment. The models used have addressed neoplasia at a number of different sites: urinary bladder, colon, intestine, kidney, liver, mammary gland, skin, and stomach, as well as sarcoma and melanoma (Tables II and III). The usual endpoint monitored in the work has been the development of hyperplasia or appearance of tumors. The effect(s) of ascorbic acid as a therapeutic agent after tumors are established, as well as in conjunction with chemotherapy and in tissue culture, have also been tested.

Bladder. Urinary bladder cancer induced in the rat by BBN, Table II, has been intensively investigated. In this model the chemical carcinogen is provided to rats in the drinking water for about 4 weeks, then they are fed a diet containing a source of vitamin C and/or other test chemical and the results are compared with a control group not receiving vitamin C or other test agent. Dietary sodium ascorbate promotes in this two-stage model, but high concentrations are required. Fukushima et al. [139] observed promotion with

5% but not 1% sodium ascorbate. As elevated urinary pH and/or Na^+ concentration were also found to promote; sodium ascorbate appears to be a copromoter [90]. Neither ascorbic acid itself nor erythrobic acid, an epimer of ascorbic acid, act as promoters, but their sodium salts enhance bladder carcinogenesis [113]. Calcium ascorbate and the ascorbate esters, L-ascorbic dipalmitate and L-ascorbate stearate, are ineffective in promotion [91]. Treatment of rats with a diet containing $NaHCO_3$ and ascorbic acid prior to initiation with carcinogen, facilitates bladder carcinogenesis [92]. Administration of $NaHCO_3$ alone to BBN-treated rats, enhances cell proliferation in the bladder, assessed by increased DNA synthesis, and promotes bladder tumor development in a dose-dependent manner. Ascorbic acid also increases bladder epithelial DNA synthesis, but has no effect on promotion. Ascorbic acid does facilitate $NaHCO_3$-promoted tumor development; thus, it appears to have an effect independent of Na^+ concentration.

The effect of sodium ascorbate on urinary bladder tumor promotion in carcinogen-initiated rats is influenced by both the rat strain studied and the diet fed. Mori et al. [93] found that although both F-344 and Lewis rats had an increased induction of lesions when initiated by BBN, the promoting effect reflected both the rat strain and the commercial diet fed. There were no differences in urinary pH or amount of Na^+, thus excluding these factors and indicating genetic factors may have a role. The potential differences in the composition of the diets fed have not been analyzed.

The effects of ascorbate on bladder cancer appear to be primarily on the promotion phase. Inoue et al. [95] tested the combined effects of L-ascorbic acid, citric acid, and their sodium salts in both the two-stage and concurrent model using BBN and EHBN [N-ethyl-N-(4-hydroxybutyl)nitrosamine] as carcinogens. In the two-stage model, both sodium ascorbate and sodium citrate have promoting activity, but have no effects when given concurrently with carcinogen. There were no differences in urinary pH or Na^+, or in the development of papillary and nodular hyperplasia between the two-stage and concurrent models.

Questions have arisen as to which animal experimental models are appropriate for investigating the relationship between ascorbic acid and chemical carcinogenesis. Humans, other primates, guinea pigs, and some birds and fishes lack L-gulonolactone oxidase activity, and are thus unable to synthesize ascorbic acid. In contrast, most other animals including rats, mice, and hamsters, species commonly used in animal cancer models, synthesize L-ascorbic acid and do not require dietary vitamin C. The guinea pig, which would seem to be the closest small animal model to humans, has not been used very extensively as a model. A recently developed rat mutant derived from the Wistar/shi rat, ODS (osteogenic disorder Shionogi, genotype: od/od [114,115]) is unable to synthesize ascorbic acid due to an autosomal, reces-

sive gene defect. Analogously with humans, the mutant has no L-gulonolactone oxidase activity and requires vitamin C as a nutrient.

Mori et al. [94] tested the responses of the ODS mutant and of ODS
heterozygotes to L-ascorbic acid using the BBN induction model. The ho-
mozygous mutant rats had a similar susceptibility to bladder cancer compared
either to heterozygotes or to normal controls, indicating that bladder cancer
is not linked with a defect in ascorbic acid synthesis. Further studies with this
promising model are indicated.

Colon. The effects of ascorbic acid on DMH-induced colon cancer in the
rat are paradoxical (Table II). Reddy et al. [96] found that dietary ascorbic
acid (2–10 g/kg) inhibited tumor development when tumors were initiated
with a single dose of DMH, but did not inhibit tumor development when
multiple doses of carcinogen were used. In contrast, Shirai et al. [98] who
fed rats a diet containing 50 g/kg of ascorbate observed enhanced tumor
development. When a commercial chow diet fed to DMH-treated rats was
supplemented with ascorbate (7% by weight), colorectal tumor incidence
(64% and 1 tumor per rat) were lower than in control rats (84% tumor
incidence and 2 tumors per rat) [59].

Gastrointestinal. The effect of vitamin C on gastrointestinal cancer has
been tested using several different carcinogens. Rats treated with MNNG
develop cancer (Table III). Although Balansky et al. [63] observed that
vitamin C reduced cancer incidence by one half as compared to controls,
Kawasaki et al. [99], in contrast, observed no effect. The antioxidant BHA
induces forestomach carcinomas in rats. In rats treated with BHA, sodium
ascorbate enhances hyperplasia in the perfundic region [65]. Sodium ascorbate also promotes tumor development in MNU-induced gastrointestinal cancer in rats [82].

Kidney. Ascorbic acid has been shown to inhibit the development of
renal cancer in several models (Table III). Kidney neoplasia in the hamster
initiated by either estradiol or DES (diethylstilbesterol) is decreased by dietary vitamin C [100]. The incidence of DMH-induced kidney tumors is also
decreased in ascorbate-treated rats [96].

Liver. Aflatoxins produce hepatic cancer in rats. The effect of ascorbic
acid on AFB (aflatoxin B_1) liver cancer is perplexing. Female Wistar rats,
pretreated with AFB and then given ascorbic acid daily for 8 months, showed
no differences in the total hepatic nodule burden as compared to controls
[101]. The ascorbate-treated group did, however, show a reduction in the
incidence of both cystic cholangiomas and hepatocellular carcinoma, but
paradoxically this group also had a significantly lower survival.

Mammary. Analyses of the effect of vitamin C on mammary neoplasia
have provided contradictory results (Table III). The occurrence of spontaneous mammary tumors in RIII mice is inhibited by vitamin C [102]. More-

over, the survival of female C3H/HEJ mice injected with mammary adeno-carcinoma cells is improved in mice receiving vitamin C as compared to controls [105]. In contrast, however, ascorbate has no effect on tumor production in DMBA-induced mammary cancer [103] while vitamin C interfered with the protective effect of dietary selenium on DMBA-induced mammary tumors in the rat [104].

Melanoma. Varga and Airoldi [106] reported that calcium ascorbate increases survival time, delays the onset of tumors, but has no effect on tumor growth in mice inoculated with melanoma cells.

Pancreas. Woutersen et al. [77] investigated the effects of vitamin C (and vitamins A and E) on pancreatic cancer induced in rats by treatment with azaserine and in hamsters by BOP. In hamsters, high vitamin C doses decreased the number of early ductal lesions observed, but the number of microcarcinomas increased. In the rat, the growth of acidophilic foci was inhibited by vitamin C.

Sarcoma. The results of vitamin C supplements on the development of sarcomas are quite variable (Table III). Ascorbate inhibits the generation of tumors in BP [benzo(a)pyrene]-treated rats [107], as well as in rats with transplanted fibrosarcoma cells [108]. Administration of vitamin C at the time of tumor implantation in the mouse reduced tumor incidence and improved survival [110]. A similar response was observed in mice inoculated with either ascitic lymphoma or lymphoblastic leukemia cells. In contrast, vitamin C evoked an increased occurrence of tumors in 3-MC (3-methylcholanthrene)-treated rats [109].

Skin. Vitamin C treatment lowered the incidence of skin cancer in ultraviolet (UV) light-treated mice [111]. Ascorbate may also have a protective role in chemical carcinogen-induced skin cancer. Smart et al. [112] tested the effects of topical applications of ascorbic acid, ascorbyl palmitate, palmitic acid, and sorbitan monopalmitate in female CD-1 mice on TPA-dependent promotion in DMBA initiated mouse skin. Ornithine decarboxylase activity, epidermal DNA synthesis, and promotion of skin tumors were assessed. Treatment with TPA resulted in an immediate, marked decrease in epidermal ascorbate. Although large doses of ascorbate prevented TPA-induced tumors; small doses did not, even though small doses of ascorbyl palmitate did inhibit ODC, DNA synthesis, and tumor promotion. Palmitic acid and sorbitan monopalmitate were less effective, but had antipromoter effects, suggesting that the effect of ascorbyl palmitate did not reflect an antioxidant effect.

Cells in culture. There is some evidence that vitamin C may facilitate growth and survival of cells in culture. The lifespan of implants of mouse and human lung carcinoma in culture were prolonged when vitamin C was added to the medium, but palmitoyl ascorbate was more effective [116]. Small amounts of vitamin C in the media suppressed the growth of human acute nonlymphocytic leukemia cells, but not of normal cells [117]. Low doses of ascorbic acid and dehydroascorbic acid enhanced cell multiplication of ascites tumor cells, whereas high doses inhibited cell proliferation [118]. Benedict et al. [119] found that the addition of ascorbate to the medium prevented the 3-MC transformation of a mouse embryo cell line.

Chemotherapy. Ascorbic acid may be beneficial as a therapeutic agent, as well as an adjunct to chemotherapy with other agents. Vitamin C had a potentiating effect in cytotoxic chemotherapy of mice with hepatomas [120]. A positive effect of ascorbate and drug treatment on melanoma in mice, however, may be manifest only when a purified diet, deficient in melanin precursor amino acids, is fed. Pierson and Meadows [121] reported that tumor growth was stimulated in melanoma-bearing mice fed a commercial diet supplemented with sodium ascorbate. In contrast, when the mice were fed the amino acid deficient, purified diet plus sodium ascorbate, tumors were smaller and animal survival was significantly higher. Treatment of the animals with the antitumor drugs (carbidopa–levodopa) had an additional beneficial effect only in mice fed the purified diet; ascorbate enhanced this effect. In contrast to the ascorbate stimulation of melanoma in chow-fed animals in the above study, Miwa et al. [116] found ascorbate had a protective effect resulting in prolongation of lifespan, not only in mice with melanoma but also with a variety of transplantable tumors (mammary, fibrosarcoma, and leukemia). In contrast, Silverman et al. [122] found no effect of vitamin C on metastases in mice bearing transplantable tumors.

VITAMIN E AND C INTERACTIONS
Synergism Between Vitamins E and C

There is a considerable amount of evidence that documents synergistic interactions between vitamins E and C. Tappel [123] was among the first to suggest that vitamin C could inhibit the oxidation of vitamin E. In vitro studies have shown that vitamin E levels are maintained by regeneration by vitamin C and that vitamins E and C cooperate in the inhibition of oxidation [10]. Niki [10] and Packer et al. [13] as well as other investigators have assessed the rates of consumption of vitamins C and E in in vitro lipid oxidizing systems and noted that initially vitamin C disappears but vitamin E levels remained constant. Subsequently, vitamin E disappeared and there was a net uptake of oxygen. Addition of vitamin C at higher concentrations afforded longer protection of vitamin E. These studies suggested that the maintenance of vitamin E concentrations and inhibition of lipid peroxidation reflected the synergistic inhibition of oxidation by vitamins C and E. The mechanism proposed is as follows: Vitamin E interaction with the lipid (L) peroxyl radical (LOO·) results in LOOH and the conversion of vitamin E to the chromonoxyl radical. This radical is in turn reduced to vitamin E by vitamin C, which is converted to the dehydroascorbate radical.

Similar effects were observed using liposomes [12,124,125], although in this system, vitamin C is not as effective.

Vitamin E is hydrophobic and a membrane component, while ascorbic acid is hydrophilic and in the soluble fraction of cells. While ascorbic acid is thus unable to directly scavenge peroxyl radicals in the membrane, it is able to regenerate the vitamin E radical. The reduction of oxidized vitamin E by a water-soluble compound such as ascorbate could occur if the phenoxyl group of vitamin E was oriented near to the water-bilayer interface. The orientation of vitamin E in membrane bilayers meets this requirement. Both nuclear magnetic resonance (NMR) studies [4] and intrinsic fluorescence analyses [126] indicate that the orientation of α-tocopherol in membranes is with the chromanol nucleus containing the phenolic hydroxyl toward the water interface of the bilayer and the phytyl side chain buried in the hydrocarbon interior of the membrane. Liebler et al. [127], however, interpreted their studies, using α-tocopherol incorporated into soybean liposomes to indicate that the pro- and antioxidant effects of ascorbic acid are determined by membrane α-tocopherol status and that ascorbic acid interacts with components of the phospholipid bilayer.

Vitamins E and C and Nitrosamines

Potential mechanisms for the postulated effect of both vitamin E and C in the protection of the development of gastrointestinal cancer may involve the blocking of nitrosamine production from nitrites and amines. A high intake of nitrates has been linked with a high incidence of stomach cancer. Nitrate can be reduced to nitrite, which can interact with other compounds to produce various N-nitroso compounds which are believed to be involved in the etiology of human cancer. Dimethylamine is synthesized by humans and even on a low nitrate intake, nitrite is present in human stomach. These nitrites can be formed in vivo both by bacterial reduction of nitrates in the gut, as well as by the action of activated macrophages [128]. The formation of N-nitroso compounds in vivo has been shown to occur in laboratory animals (140). Direct evidence that nitrosamines are synthesized by humans following the ingestion of an amine (proline) and nitrate has been obtained by monitoring the urinary excretion of N-nitrosoproline [129].

In systems in which the formation of N-nitroso compounds is inhibited, carcinogenic action is blocked. Vitamins E [130] and C [131] block nitrosamine formation. These vitamins appear to act by competing with susceptible amines and amides for the nitrosating agent, which, by acting as antioxidants, they reduce to a nonnitrosating compound. Dehydroascorbic acid and tocopherol quinone are the products of the reaction of vitamins C and E, respectively, with a nitrosating agent.

Vitamins E and C have been shown to inhibit nitroso compound initiated cancer in animal studies. Many early animal studies concerned the effect of dietary treatment with tocopherol or ascorbic acid on the carcinogenicity of nitroso compounds [132–135]. *N*-Nitroso induction of lung cancer was inhibited in mice treated with ascorbic acid [136]. Administration of either vitamin E or C protected rats from the hepatotoxicity caused by dimethylnitrosamine (DMN), which was formed by feeding nitrite and aminopyrene [137].

A variety of nitrosamine compounds (BBN, DMH, and MNNG) are effective inducers of cancer in animal models (Tables I–III). Interpretation of the effects of vitamins E and C in these models is very challenging. Even when an apparently identical model is used in different studies to test the effectiveness of tocopherol and ascorbic acid, the experimental procedures often vary. In many studies diet supplementation involves additions of the vitamins to a commercial chow, rather than to a purified diet. Many of the species used synthesize ascorbic acid and in most cases begin the study with adequate vitamin E. Given such limitations and assuming the study protocols are analogous, studies of the comparative effects of tocopherol and ascorbate treatments in the following rat–nitroso cancer models have been made: BBN–bladder, DMH–colon, MNNG–gastric, and the hamster BOP–pancreas model. The results obtained are quite variable. Sodium ascorbate promotes rather than inhibits BBN-initiated bladder cancer; vitamin E has no effect. Vitamins E and C are both reported to decrease DMN-induced colon tumors and also to have no effect. The same spectrum of effects occurs in MNNG-induced gastrointestinal neoplasia. In the pancreatic model, ascorbate inhibited while vitamin E had no effect. Although vitamins C and E both modulate nitroso-induced carcinogenesis in the rat, a simple generalization is difficult to make. Obviously, development of carcinogenesis is very complex and each nitroso compound and model are unique. This may explain the diversity and contradictory nature of the results obtained.

As with the experimental animal studies, the results of epidemiological studies are not consistent. They do, however, suggest there may be a correlation between intake of vitamins E and C, as reflected by serum concentrations, and the risk for certain types of cancer. Stähelin et al. [28], in the Basel study, observed that subjects with low vitamin C and low vitamin E had an increased gastrointestinal cancer mortality risk, suggesting there may be a synergism between them.

Vitamins E and C and Other Carcinogens

Other models in which vitamins E and C have both been tested include DMBA-induced rat mammary cancer (Tables I and III). Vitamin E has no protective effect in this model, but does enhance the inhibition of tumor development by selenium; vitamin C interferes with this effect. In contrast, in the two-stage DMBA-initiated mouse skin cancer model, both vitamins E and C are inhibitory (Tables I and III).

POTENTIAL MECHANISMS

It is quite clear from in vitro studies that the chemical properties of vitamins E and C predict that they would be effective anticancer agents, and that there are interactions between α-tocopherol and ascorbic acid. Human epidemiological studies indirectly implicate a protective role for these vitamins. Studies in experimental animals document that vitamins E and C do appear to influence the process of tumorigenesis, but the reported effects tend to be conflicting. The in vitro effects of vitamins E and C on nitrosamines, are not unambiguously documented in animal models. Moreover, analyses using other carcinogens and transplantable tumors, although showing effects of these vitamins also are fraught with contradictory results. Nonetheless, in spite of these problems, taken together the evidence that vitamins E and C have a role in neoplasia is reasonably firm. The mechanisms for the observed effects have not been clarified.

Oxidative stress and cellular immunity both appear to have important roles in cancer and both vitamins E and C have effects on them. The body defense potential in cancer is related to endogenous antioxidant defense systems and the status of antioxidant vitamins. That vitamin E protects cells from injury due to oxidative stress is well documented. Isolated rat hepatocytes grown in the absence of Ca^{2+} provide a model of oxidative stress responsive to vitamin E [138]. An early event in this model is loss of cellular α-tocopherol associated with a change in the structure of the plasma membrane, followed by lipid peroxidation and efflux of glutathione. The mechanisms of stress and protective effect of vitamin E in this model include membrane structure changes and free radical scavenging by vitamin E. Specific molecular species within phospholipid classes may be precursors of biological mediators and are closely associated with membrane receptors. The precise localization of vitamin E within a specific membrane phosphatide domain is not known. Protein–lipid interactions affect protein functions. Membrane-bound enzymes and proteins require a lipid bilayer to be functional; lipid peroxidation alters the bilayer. Membrane-resident vitamin E has a role in the modulation of membrane function and may be an integral part of the receptor-activated cascade of reactions regulating the biology of cells.

Carcinogenesis is a complex multistage process. Factors that influence cancer development may have an effect on carcinogen activation, initiation, and promotion. In several of the models, vitamins E and C exert their effects during the promotion phase. The requirements for tumor growth and development include many factors including cell regulators. Vitamins E and C may function in the regulation of such growth factors. Further information on the mechanisms of function of vitamins C and E at the molecular cellular level will be essential for understanding their role(s) and potential interactions in cell biology and in cancer.

REFERENCES

1. Hochstein P, Atallah AS (1988): The nature of oxidants and antioxidant systems in the inhibition of mutation and cancer. Mutation Res 202:363–375.
2. Tappel AL (1962): Vitamin E as the biological lipid oxidant. Vitamin Horm 20:493–510.
3. Diplock AT, Lucy JA (1973): The biochemical modes of action of vitamin E and selenium: a hypothesis. FEBS Lett 29:205–210.
4. Perly B, Smith IC, Hughes L, Burton GW, Ingold KU (1985): Estimation of the location of natural α-tocopherol in lipid bilayers by ^{13}C-NMR spectroscopy. Biochim Biophys Acta 819:131–135.
5. Erin AN, Skrypin VV, Kagan VE (1985): Formation of α-tocopherol complexes with fatty acid: nature of complexes. Biochim Biophys Acta 815:209–214.
6. Urano S, Iida M, Otani I, Matuo M (1987): Membrane stabilization of vitamin E: interactions of α-tocopherol with phospholipids in bilayer liposomes. Biochem Biophys Res Commun 146:1413–1418.
7. Steiner M (1981): Vitamin E changes the membrane fluidity of human platelets. Biochim Biophys Acta 640:100–105.
8. Ohyashiki T, Ushiro H, Mohri T (1986): Effects of α-tocopherol on the lipid peroxidation and fluidity of porcine intestinal brush-border membranes. Biochim Biophys Acta 858: 294–300.
9. Moran J, Salazar P, Pasantes-Morales H (1987): Effect of tocopherol and taurine on membrane fluidity of retinal rod outer segments. Exp Eye Res 45:769–776.
10. Niki E (1987): Interaction of ascorbate and α-tocopherol. Ann NY Acad Sci 498:186–199.
11. Mukai K, Nishimura M, Ishizu K, Kitamura Y (1989): Kinetic study of the reaction of vitamin C with vitamin E radicals, tocopheroxyls, in solution. Biochim Biophys Acta 991:276–279.
12. Scarpa M, Rigo A, Maioring M, Ursini F, Gregolin C (1984): Formation of α-tocopherol radical and recycling of α-tocopherol by ascorbate during peroxidation of phosphatidylcholine by liposomes. An electron paramagnetic resonance study. Biochim Biophys Acta 801:215–219.
13. Packer JE, Slater TF, Willson RL (1979): Direct observation of a free radical interaction between vitamin E and vitamin C. Nature 278:737–738.
14. Morre F, Crane L, Sun IL, Navas P (1987): The role of ascorbate in biomembrane energetics. Ann NY Acad Sci 498:153–179.
15. Schwarz RI, Kleinman P, Owens N (1987): Ascorbate can act as an inducer of the collagen pathway because most steps are tightly coupled. Ann NY Acad Sci 498:172–185.
16. Glembowski CC (1987): The role of ascorbic acid in the biosynthesis of the neuropeptides α-MSH and TRH. Ann NY Acad Sci 498:54–62.

17. Salonen JT, Salonen R, Lappetelainen R, Maenpaa PH, Alfithan G, Puska P (1985): Risk of cancer in relation to serum concentrations of vitamins A and E: Matched case control analyses of prospective data. Br Med J 290:417–420.
18. Stähelin HB, Rosel F, Buess E, Brubacher G (1984): Cancer, vitamins, and plasma lipids: Prospective Basel study. J Natl Cancer Inst 73:1463–1468.
19. Willett WC, Polk BF, Junderwood BA, Stampfer MJ, Presel S, Rosner B, Taylor JO, Schneider K, Hames CG (1984): Relation of serum vitamins A and E and carotenoids to the risk of cancer. N Engl J Med 310:430–434.
20. Nomura AMY, Stennermann GN, Heilbrun LK, Salkeld RM, Vuilleumier JP (1985): Serum vitamin levels and the risk of cancer of specific sites in men of Japanese ancestry in Hawaii. Cancer Res 45:2369–2372.
21. Wald NJ, Thompson SG, Densem JW, Boreham J, Bailey A (1987): Serum vitamin E and subsequent risk of cancer. Br J Cancer 56:69–72.
22. Wald NJ, Boreham J, Hayward JL, Bulbrook RD (1984): Plasma retinol, beta carotene, and vitamin E levels in relation to the future risk of breast cancer. Br J Cancer 49: 321–324.
23. Wald NJ, Nicolaides-Bouman A, Hudson GA (1988): Letter to the editor. Plasma retinol, beta-carotene and vitamin E levels in relation to the future risk of breast cancer. Br J Cancer 57:235.
24. Russell MJ, Thomas BS, Bulbrook RD (1988): A prospective study of the relationship between serum vitamins A and E and risk of breast cancer. Br J Cancer 57:213–215.
25. Heinonen PK, Kosinen T, Tuimala AR (1985): Serum levels of vitamins A and E in women with ovarian cancer. Arch Gynecol 237:37–40.
26. Gerber M, Cavallo F, Marubini E, Richardon S, Barbieri A, Capitelli AC, DePaulet AC, DePaulet PC, Decarli A, Pastorino U, Pujol H (1988): Liposoluble vitamins and lipid parameters in breast cancer. A joint study in northern Italy and southern France. Int J Cancer 42:489–494.
27. Langemann H, Torhorst J, Kabiersch A, Krenger W, Honegger CG (1989): Quantitative determination of water- and lipid-soluble antioxidants in neoplastic and non-neoplastic human breast tissue. Int J Cancer 43:1169–1173.
28. Stähelin HB, Gey KF, Brubacher G (1987): Plasma vitamin C and cancer death: The Basel study. Ann NY Acad Sci 498:124–131.
29. Gey KFG, Brubacher GB, Stähelin HB (1987): Plasma levels of antioxidant vitamins in relation to ischemic heart disease and cancer. Am J Clin Nutr 45:1368–1377.
30. Knekt P (1988): Serum vitamin E level and risk of female cancers. Int J Epidemiol 17:281–288.
31. Knekt P, Aromaa A, Maatela J, Alfthan G, Aaran R, Teppo L, Hakama M (1988): Serum vitamin E, serum selenium and the risk of gastrointestinal cancer. Int J Cancer 42: 846–850.
32. Knekt P, Aromaa A, Maatela J, Aaran R, Nikkari T, Hakama M, Hakulinen T, Peto R, Sacen E, Teppo L (1988): Serum vitamin E and risk of cancer among Finnish men during a 10-year follow-up. Am J Epidemiol 127:28–41.
33. Sundström HK, Sajanti E, Kauppila A (1989): Supplementation with selenium, vitamin E and their combination on gynaecological cancer during cytotoxic chemotherapy. Carcinogenesis 10:273–278.
34. Stähelin HB, Gey KF, Eicholzer M, Ludin E, Brubacher G (1989): Cancer mortality and vitamin E status. Ann NY Acad Sci 570:391–399.
35. Menkes MS, Constock GW, Vuillemier JP, Helsing KJ, Rider AA, Brookmeyer R (1986): Serum beta-carotene, vitamins A and E, selenium and the risk of lung cancer. N Engl J Med 315:1250–1254.

36. Kok FJ, Duijn CM, Hofman A, Vermeeren R, Debruijn AM, Valenburg HA (1987): Micronutrients and the risk of lung cancer. N Engl J Med 316:1416.
37. Miyamoto H, Araya Y, Ito M, Isobe H, Dosaka H, Shimizu T, Kishi F, Yamamoto I, Honma H, Kawakami Y (1987): Serum selenium and vitamin E concentrations in families of lung cancer patients. Cancer 60:1159–1162.
38. Hormozdiari H, Day NE, Aramesh B, Mahboubi E (1975): Dietary factors and esophageal cancer in the Caspian littoral of Iran. Cancer Res 35:3493–3498.
39. Mettlin C, Graham S, Priore R, Swanson M (1981): Diet and cancer of the esophagus. Nutr Cancer 2:143–147.
40. Cook-Mozaffari P, Azzordegan F, Day NE, Ressicand A, Sabai C, Aramesh B (1979): The epidemiology of cancer of the esophagus. Nutr Cancer 1:51–60.
41. Yang CS, Sun Y, Yang QU, Miller KW, Li GY, Cheng SF (1984): Vitamin A and other deficiencies in Linxian, a high esophageal cancer incidence area in northern China. J Natl Cancer Inst 73:1449–1453.
42. Higginson J (1966): Etiological factors in gastro-intestinal cancer in man. J Natl Cancer Inst 37:527–545.
43. Graham S, Dayal H, Swanson M, Nittelman A, Wilkinson G (1978): Diet in the epidemiology of cancer of the colon and rectum. J Natl Cancer Inst 61:709–714.
44. Jain M, Cook GM, Davis FG, Grace MG, Howe GR, Miller AB (1980): A case control study of diet and colorectal cancer. Int J Cancer 26:757–76.
45. Fontham ETH, Pickle LW, Haenszel W, Correa P, Lin Y, Falk RT (1988): Dietary vitamins A and C and lung cancer risk in Louisiana. Cancer 62:2267–2273.
46. Hinds MW, Kolonel LN (1984): Dietary vitamin A, carotene, vitamin C and risk of lung cancer in Hawaii. Am J Epidemiol 119:227–237.
47. Byers TE, Graham S, Haughey BP, Marshall JR, Swanson MK (1987): Diet and lung cancer risk: Findings from the western New York diet study. Am J Epidemiol 125:351–363.
48. Marshall J, Graham S, Mettlin C, Shedd G, Swanson M (1982): Diet in the epidemiology of oral cancer. Nutr Cancer 3:145–149.
49. Graham S, Mettlin C, Marshall J, Priore R, Rzepka T, Shedd D (1981): Dietary factors in the epidemiology of cancer of the larynx. Am J Epidemiol 113:675–680.
50. Cameron E, Pauling L (1976): Supplemental ascorbate in the supportive treatment of cancer: Prolongation of survival times in terminal human cancer. Proc Natl Acad Sci USA 73:3685–3689.
51. Creagan ET, Moertal GG, O'Fallon JR, Schutt AJ, O'Connell MJ, Rubin J, Frytak S (1979): Failure of high-dose vitamin C therapy to benefit patients with advanced cancer. A control trial. N Engl J Med 301:687–690.
52. Moertel CG, Fleming TR, Creagan ET, Rubin J, O'Connell MJ, Ames M (1985): High-dose vitamin C versus placebo in the treatment of patients with advanced cancer who have had no prior chemotherapy. A randomized double-blind study. N Engl J Med 312:137–141.
53. McKeown-Eyssen G, Holloway C, Bright-See E, Dion P, Bruce WR (1988): A randomized trial of vitamins C and E in the prevention of recurrence of colorectal polyps. Cancer Res 48:4701–4705.
54. DeCosse JJ (1982): Potential for chemoprevention. Cancer 50:2550–2553.
55. Moriarty MJ, Mulgrew S, Malone JF, O'Connor MK (1977): Results and analysis of tumor levels of ascorbic acid. Irish J Med Sci 146:74–78.
56. Moriarty M, Mulgrew S, Mothersill C, Malone JF, Hatch M (1978): Some effects of administration of large doses of vitamin C in patients with skin carcinoma. Irish J Med Sci 147:166–170.

57. Marcus SL, Dutcher JP, Paietta E, Ciobanu N, Strauman J, Wiernik PH, Hutner SH, Frank O, Baker H (1987): Severe hypovitaminosis C occurring as the result of adoptive immunotherapy with high-dose interleukin 2 and lymphokine-activated killer cells. Cancer Res 47:4208–4212.

58. Tamano S, Fukushima S, Shirai T, Hirose M, Ito N (1987): Modification by α-tocopherol, propyl gallate and tertiary butylhydroquinone of urinary bladder carcinogenesis in Fisher 344 rats pretreated with N-butyl-N-(4-hydroxybutyl)nitrosamine. Cancer Lett 35: 39–46.

59. Colacchio TA, Memoli VA, Hildebrandt L (1989): Antioxidants vs carotenoids. Inhibitors or promoters of experimental colorectal cancers. Arch Surg 124:217–221.

60. Slater G, Kang J, Cohen G, Szporn A, Aufses AH (1987): In vivo ethane production in vitamin E-deficient rats with DMH-induced colon cancer. J Surg Oncol 36:142–147.

61. Cook MG, McNamara P (1980): Effect of dietary vitamin E on dimethylhydrazine-induced colonic tumors in mice. Cancer Res 40:1329–1331.

62. Toth B, Patil K (1983): Enhancing effect of vitamin E on murine intestinal tumorigenesis by 1,2-dimethylhydrazine dihydrochloride. J Natl Cancer Inst 70:1107–1111.

63. Balansky RM, Blagoeva PM, Mircheva ZI, Stoitchev I, Chernozemski I (1986): The effect of antioxidants on MNNG-induced stomach carcinogenesis in rats. J Cancer Res Clin Oncol 112:272–275.

64. Takahashi M, Furukawa F, Toyoda K, Sato H, Hasegawa R, Hayashi Y (1986): Effects of four antioxidants on N-methyl-N'-nitro-N-nitrosoguanidine initiated gastric tumor development in rats. Cancer Lett 30:161–166.

65. Hirose M, Masuda A, Tsuda H, Awagawa S, Ito N (1987): Enhancement of BHA-induced proliferative rat forestomach lesion development by simultaneous treatment with other antioxidants. Carcinogenesis 8:1731–1735.

66. Ura H, Denda A, Yokose Y, Tsutsumi M, Konishi Y (1987): Effect of vitamin E on the induction and evolution of enzyme-altered foci in the liver of rats treated with diethylnitrosamine. Carcinogenesis 8:1595–1600.

67. Moore MA, Tsuda H, Thamavit W, Masui T, Ito N (1987): Differential modification of development of preneoplastic lesions in the Syrian golden hamster initiated with a single dose of 2,2'-dioxo-N-nitrosopropylamine: influence of subsequent butylated hydroxyanisole, α-tocopherol, or carbazole. J Natl Cancer Inst 78:289–292.

68. Ip C (1982): Dietary vitamin E intake and mammary carcinogenesis in rats. Carcinogenesis 3:1453–1456.

69. Horvath PM, Ip C (1983): Synergistic effect of vitamin E and selenium in the chemoprevention of mammary carcinogenesis in rats. Cancer Res 43:5335–5341.

70. King MM, McCay PB (1983): Modulation of tumor incidence and possible mechanism of inhibition of mammary carcinogenesis by dietary antioxidants. Cancer Res 43:2485s–2490s.

71. Ip C, White G (1987): Mammary cancer chemoprevention by inorganic and organic selenium: Single agent treatment or in combination with vitamin E and their effects on in vitro immune functions. Carcinogenesis 8:1763–1766.

72. Beth M, Berger MR, Aksoy M, Schmähl D (1987): Effects of vitamin A and E supplementation to diets containing two different fat levels on methylnitrosourea-induced mammary carcinogenesis in female SD-rats vitamin E-cancer. Br J Cancer 56:445–449.

73. Shklar G (1982): Oral mucosal carcinogenesis in hamsters: Inhibition by vitamin E. J Natl Cancer Inst 68:791–797.

74. Trickler D, Shklar G (1987): Prevention by vitamin E of experimental oral carcinogenesis. J Natl Cancer Inst 78:165–169.

75. Shklar G, Schwartz J (1988): Tumor necrosis factor in experimental cancer: Regression with α-tocopherol, beta-carotene, canthaxanthin and algae extract. Eur J Cancer Clin Oncol 24:839–850.
76. Calhoun KH, Stanley D, Stiernberg M (1989): Vitamins A and E do protect against oral carcinoma. Arch Otolaryngol Head Neck Surg 115:484–488.
77. Woutersen RA, van Garderen-Hoetmer A (1988): Inhibition of dietary fat-promoted development of (pre)neoplastic lesions in exocrine pancreas of rats and hamsters by supplemental vitamins A, C and E. Cancer Lett 41:179–189.
78. Perchellet J, Owen MD, Posey TD, Orten DK, Schneider BA (1985): Inhibitory effects of glutathione level-raising agents and D-L-α-tocopherol on ornithine decarboxylase induction and mouse skin tumor promotion by 12-*O*-tetradecanoylphorbol-13-acetate. Carcinogenesis 6:567–573.
79. Perchellet J, Abney NL, Thomas RM, Guislain YL, Perchellet E (1987): Effects of combined treatments with selenium, glutathione, and vitamin E on glutathione peroxidase activity, ornithine decarboxylase induction and complete and multistage carcinogenesis in mouse skin. Cancer Res 47:477–485.
80. Rotstein JB, Slaga TJ (1988): Effect of exogenous glutathione on tumor progression in the murine multistage carcinogenesis model. Carcinogenesis 9:1547–1551.
81. Imaida K, Fukushima S, Shirai T, Ohtani M, Nakanishi K, Ito N (1983): Promoting activities of butylated hydroxyanisole and butylated hydroxytoluene on 2-stage urinary bladder carcinogenesis and inhibition of gamma-glutamyl transpeptidase positive foci development in the liver of rats. Carcinogenesis 4:895–899.
82. Imaida K, Fukushima S, Shirai T, Masui T, Ogiso T, Ito N (1984): Promoting activities of butylated hydroxyanisole, butylated hydroxytoluene and sodium l-ascorbate on forestomach and urinary bladder carcinogenesis initiated with methylnitrosourea in F344 male rats. Gann 75:769–775.
83. Hirose M, Fukushima S, Kurata Y, Tsuda H, Tatematsu M, Ito N (1988): Modification of *N*-methyl-*N'*-nitro-*N*-nitrosoguanidine-induced forestomach and glandular stomach carcinogenesis by phenolic antioxidants in rats. Cancer Res 48:5310–5315.
84a. Cheeseman KH, Collins M, Proudfoot K, Slater TF, Burton GW, Webb AC, Ingold KU (1986): Studies on lipid peroxidation in normal and tumour tissues. The Novikoff rat liver tumour. Biochem J 235:507–514.
84b. Cheeseman KH, Emery S, Maddix SP, Slater TF, Burton GW, Ingold KU (1988): Studies on lipid peroxidation in normal and tumour tissues. The Yoshida rat liver tumour. Biochem J 250:247–252.
85. Odukoya O, Hawach F, Shklar G (1984): Retardation of experimental oral cancer by topical vitamin E. Nutr Cancer 6:98–104.
86. Schwartz J, Suda D, Light G (1986): Beta-carotene is associated with the regression of hamster buccal pouch carcinoma and the induction of tumor necrosis factor in macrophages. Biochem Biophys Res Commun 136:1130–1135.
87. Borek C, Ong A, Mason H, Donahue L, Biaglow JE (1986): Selenium and vitamin E inhibit radiogenic and chemically induced transformation *in vitro* via different mechanisms of action. Proc Natl Acad Sci USA 83:1490–1494.
88. Weitberg B (1987): Effects of inhibitors of arachidonic acid metabolism and vitamin E on oxygen radical-induced sister chromatid exchanges. Carcinogenesis 8:1619–1620.
89. Odukoya O, Schwartz J, Shklar G (1986): Vitamin E stimulates proliferation of experimental oral carcinoma cells *in vitro*. Nutr Cancer 8:101–106.
90. Fukushima S, Shibata MA, Shirai T, Tamano S, Ito N (1986): Roles of urinary sodium ion concentration and pH in promotion by ascorbic acid of urinary bladder carcinogenesis in rat. Cancer Res 46:1623–1626.

91. Fukushima S, Ogiso T, Kurata Y, Shibata M, Kakizoe T (1987): Absence of promotion potential for calcium l-ascorbate, l-ascorbic dipalmitate, l-ascorbic stearate and erythrobic acid on rat urinary bladder carcinogenesis. Cancer Lett 35:17–25.
92. Fukushima S, Imaida K, Shibata M, Tamono S, Kurata Y, Shirai T (1988): L-Ascorbic acid amplification of second-stage bladder carcinogenesis promotion by $NaHCO_3$. Cancer Res 48:6317–6320.
93. Mori S, Kurata Y, Takeuchi T, Toyama M, Makino S, Fukushima S (1987): Influences of strain and diet on the promoting effects of sodium l-ascorbate in two-stage urinary bladder carcinogenesis in rats. Cancer Res 47:3492–3495.
94. Mori S, Takeuchi Y, Toyama M, Makino S, Harauchi T, Kurata Y, Fukushima S (1988): Assessment of l-ascorbic acid requirement for prolonged survival in ODS rats and their susceptibility to urinary bladder carcinogenesis by N-butyl-N-(4-hydroxybutyl)nitrosamine. Cancer Lett 38:275–282.
95. Inoue T, Katsumi I, Suzuki E, Okada M, Fukushima S (1988): Combined effects of l-ascorbic acid, citric acid or their sodium salts on tumor induction by N-butyl-N-(4-hydroxybutyl)nitrosamine or N-ethyl-N(4-hydroxybutyl)nitrosamine in the rat urinary bladder. Cancer Lett 40:265–273.
96. Reddy BS, Hiroto N, Katayame S (1982): Effect of dietary sodium ascorbate on 1,2-dimethylhydrazine-induced colon carcinogenesis in rats. Carcinogenesis 3:1097–1099.
97. Colacchio TA, Memoli VA (1986): Chemoprevention of colorectal neoplasms. Arch Surg 121:1421–1424.
98. Shirai T, Ikawa E, Hirose M, Thamavit W, Ito N (1985): Modification by five antioxidants of 1,2-dimethylhydrazine-induced colon carcinogenesis in F344 rats. Carcinogenesis 6:637–639.
99. Kawasaki H, Morishinge F, Tanaka H, Kimoto E (1982): Influence of oral supplementation of ascorbate upon the induction of N-methyl-N'-nitro-N-nitrosoguanidine. Cancer Lett 41:1425–1430.
100. Liehr JG, Wheeler WJ (1983): Inhibition of estrogen-induced renal carcinoma in Syrian hamsters by vitamin C. Cancer Res 43:4638–4642.
101. Iverson F, Campbell J, Clayson D, Hierlihy S, Labossiere E, Hayward S (1987): Effects of antioxidants on Aflatoxin-induced hepatic tumors in rats. Cancer Lett:139–144.
102. Pauling L, Nixon JC, Stit F, Marcuson R, Dunham WB, Barth R, Bensch R, Herman ZS, Blaisdell BE, Tsao C (1985): Effect of dietary ascorbic acid on the incidence of spontaneous mammary tumors in RIII mice. Proc Natl Acad Sci USA 82:5185–5189.
103. Abul-Hajj YJ, Kelliher M (1982): Failure of ascorbic acid to inhibit growth of transplantable and dimethylbenzanthracene-induced rat mammary tumors. Cancer Lett 17:67–83.
104. Ip C (1986): Interaction of vitamin C and selenium supplementation in the modification of mammary carcinogenesis in rats. J Natl Cancer Inst 77:299–303.
105. Frazier T, McGinn M (1979): The influence of magnesium, calcium, and vitamin C on tumor growth in mice with breast cancer. J Surg Res 27:318–320.
106. Varga JM, Airdoli L (1983): Inhibition of transplantable melanoma tumor development in mice by prophylactic administration of Ca-ascorbate. Life Sci 32:1559–1564.
107. Kallistratos G, Fasske E (1980): Inhibition of benzo(a)pyrene carcinogenesis in rats with vitamin C. J Cancer Res Clin Oncol 97:91–96.
108. Kallistratos G, Fasske E (1983): The effect of vitamin C on transplanted fibrosarcoma cells in rats. J Med Sci 1:9–12.
109. Banic S (1981): Vitamin C acts as a cocarcinogen to methylcholanthrene in guinea-pigs. Cancer Lett 11:139–142.

110. Ghosh J, Das S (1985): Evaluation of vitamin A and C status in normal and malignant conditions and their possible role in cancer prevention. Jpn J Cancer Res 76:1174–2278.
111. Dunham WB, Zukerhandle E, Reynolds R (1982): Effects of intake of l-ascorbic acid on the incidence of dermal neoplasms induced in mice by ultraviolet light. Proc Natl Acad Sci USA 79:7532–7536.
112. Smart RC, Huang MT, Han ZT, Kaplan MC, Focella A, Conney AH (1987): Inhibition of 12-*O*-tetradecanoylphorbol-12-acetate induction of ornithine decarboxylase activity, DNA synthesis, and tumor promotion in mouse skin by ascorbic acid and ascorbyl palmitate. Cancer Res 47:6633–6638.
113. Fukushima S, Kurata Y, Shibata MA, Ikawa E, Ito N (1984): Promotion by ascorbic acid, sodium erythrobate and ethoxyquin of neoplastic lesions in rats initiated with *N*-butyl-*N*-(4-hydroxylbutyl)nitrosamine. Cancer Lett 23:4454–4457.
114. Mitzushima Y, Harauchi T, Yoshizaki T, Makino S (1984): A rat mutant unable to synthesize vitamin C. Experientia 40:259–361.
115. Horio F, Ozaki K, Yoshida A, Makino S, Hayashi Y (1985): Ascorbic acid requirement in a rat mutant unable to synthesize ascorbic acid. J Nutr 115:1630–1640.
116. Miwa N, Yamazaki H, Nagaoka Y, Kageyama K, Onoyama Y, Matusi-Yuasa I, Otani S, Morisawa S (1986): Altered production of the active species is involved in enhanced cytotoxic action of acylated derivatives of ascorbate to tumor cells. Biochim Biophys Acta 972:144–151.
117. Park CH, Amare M, Savin MA, Hoogstraten B (1980): Growth suppression of human leukemic cells *in vitro* by l-ascorbic acid. Cancer Res 40:1062–1065.
118. Liotti FS, Menghini AR, Guerrieri P, Talesa V, Bodo M (1984): Effects of ascorbic acid and dehydroascorbic acid on the multiplication of tumor ascites cells *in vitro*. J Cancer Res Clin Oncol 108:230–232.
119. Benedict WF, Wheatley WL, Jones PA (1980): Inhibition of chemically induced morphological transformation and reversion of the transformed phenotype by ascorbic acid in C3H/10T-1/3 cells. Cancer Res 40:2796–2801.
120. Taper HS, De Gerlache J, Lans M, Roberfroid M (1987): The toxic potentiation of cancer chemotherapy by combined C and K$_3$ vitamin pretreatment. Cancer 40:575–579.
121. Pierson HF, Meadows GG (1983): Sodium ascorbate enhancement of carbidopa-levodopa ester antitumor activity against pigmented B16 melanoma. Cancer Res 43:2017–2051.
122. Silverman J, Rivenson A, Reddy B (1983): Effect of sodium ascorbate on transplantable murine tumors. Nutr Cancer 4:192–197.
123. Tappel AL (1968): Will antioxidant nutrients slow the aging process? Geriatrics 23:97–105.
124. Niki E, Kawakami Y, Yamamoto Y, Kamiya Y (1985): Synergistic inhibition of oxidation of soybean phosphatidylcholine liposomes in aqueous dispersion by vitamin E and vitamin C. Bull Chem Soc Jpn 58:1971–1975.
125. Doba TG, Burton GW, Ingold KU (1985): Antioxidant and co-oxidant activity of vitamin C. The effect of vitamin C either alone or in the presence of vitamin E or a water-soluble vitamin E analogue, upon the peroxidation of multilamellar phospholipid liposomes. Biochim Biophys Acta 835:235–303.
126. Kagen VE, Quinn PJ (1988): The interaction of α-tocopherol and homologues with shorter hydrocarbon chains with phospholipid bilayer dispersions. A fluorescence probe study. Eur J Biochem 171:661–667.
127. Liebler DC, Kling DS, Reed DJ (1986): Antioxidant protection of phospholipid bilayers by α-tocopherol. Control of α-tocopherol status and lipid peroxidation by ascorbic acid and glutathione. J Biol Chem 261:12114–12119.

128. Tannenbaum SR, Wishnok JS (1987): Inhibition of nitrosamine formation by ascorbic acid. Ann NY Acad Sci 498:354–363.
129. Ohshima H, Bartsch H (1981): Quantitative estimation of endogenous nitrosation in humans by monitoring *N*-nitrosoproline excreted in the urine. Cancer Res 41:3658–3662.
130. Mergens WJ (1982): Effect of vitamin E to prevent nitrosamine formation. Ann NY Acad Sci 393:61–69.
131. Mirvish SS, Wallcave L, Eagen M, Shubik P (1972): Ascorbate–nitrate reaction: Possible means of blocking the formation of carcinogenic *N*-nitroso compounds. Science 177: 65–68.
132. Birt D (1986): Update on the effects of vitamins A, C and E and selenium on carcinogenesis. Proc Soc Exp Biol Med 183:311–320.
133. Chen LH, Boissonneault GA, Glauert HP (1988): Vitamin C, vitamin E and cancer. Anticancer Res 8:739–748.
134. National Academy of Sciences, National Research Council (1982): Diet, nutrition and cancer. National Academy Press, Washington DC.
135. Newberne PM, Suphakarn V (1983): Nutrition and cancer: A review, with emphasis on the role of vitamins C and E and selenium. Nutr Cancer 5:109–119.
136. Mirvish SS, Cardesa A, Wallcave L, Shubik P (1975): Induction of mouse lung adenomas by amines or urea plus nitrite and by *N*-nitroso compounds: Effect of ascorbate, gallic acid, thiocyanate, and caffeine. J Natl Cancer Inst 55:633–636.
137. Kamm JJT, Dashman T, Conney AH, Burns JJ (1973): Protective action of ascorbic acid on hepatotoxicity caused by nitrite plus aminopyrene. Proc Natl Acad Sci USA 70: 747–749.
138. Pascoe GA, Reed DJ (1989): Cell calcium, vitamin E, and the thiol redox system in cytotoxicity. Free Radical Biology and Medicine 6:209–224.
139. Fukushima S, Imaida K, Sakata T, Shibata M, Ito N (1983): Promoting effect of sodium-ascorbate on two-stage bladder carcinogenesis in rats. Cancer Res 43:4454–4457.
140. Mirvish, SS, Karlowski K, Birt DF, Sams JP (1980): Dietary and other factors affecting nitrosomethyurea (NMU) formation in the rat stomach. In Walker EA, Griciute L, Castegnaro M, Borzonyi M, Davis W, (eds): "N-Nitroso Compounds: Analysis formation and occurrence." IARC Scientific Publications No. 32. Lyon, France: International Agency for Research on Cancer, pp 271–277.

Vitamins and Cancer Prevention, pages 91–102
© *1991 Wiley-Liss, Inc.*

7 | 1,25-Dihydroxyvitamin D₃ and Hematopoietic Cells: Applications to Cancer Therapy

Masahiro Kizaki, M.D.
H. Phillip Koeffler, M.D.

INTRODUCTION

The active form of vitamin D_3 is 1,25-dihydroxyvitamin D_3 [$1,25(OH)_2D_3$], which results from sequential hydroxylation in the liver and kidney. The $1,25(OH)_2D_3$ is generally accepted as the principal form of vitamin D_3 responsible for calcium homeostasis in humans [1–3]. The classic target organs of this seco-steroid are the intestine, bone, and kidney. Recently, the vitamin D_3 endocrine system was found to interact with the hematopoietic system. The evidence for these interactions includes the following:

1. Hematopoietic cells have receptors for $1,25(OH)_2D_3$.

Department of Medicine, Division of Hematology–Oncology, University of California at Los Angeles, Los Angeles, California 90024

2. The $1,25(OH)_2D_3$ modulates differentiation of the myeloid stem cell known as the colony-forming unit granulocyte–macrophage (CFU–GM) towards macrophages [4,5].

3. Low concentrations of $1,25(OH)_2D_3$ induce neoplastic cells from several myeloid cell lines (HL-60, U937) to differentiate to macrophagelike cells [6–9].

4. Activated normal macrophages can synthesize $1,25(OH)_2D_3$ [10].

Acute myelogenous leukemia (AML) arises from neoplastic transformation of a myeloid stem cell, leading to a block in cellular maturation at the myeloblast or promyelocyte stage. Many of the leukemic cells remain in the proliferative pool and rapidly accumulate. The leukemic patients often die of infection because the blast cells cannot mature to functional-end cells. One possible approach to treatment of these patients is to induce differentiation and/or to inhibit clonal proliferation of their leukemic cells, thereby eliminating these cells from the proliferative pool. Clonogenic blast cells from patients with AML are inhibited in their proliferation by $1,25(OH)_2D_3$ [5]. Studies in vivo also suggest that $1,25(OH)_2D_3$ can prolong the survival of mice injected with leukemic cells [11]. In this chapter we will discuss the role of $1,25(OH)_2D_3$ in the hematopoietic system.

EFFECTS OF $1,25(OH)_2D_3$ ON NORMAL AND LEUKEMIC MYELOID CELLS IN VITRO

A diagram of the human hematopoietic system with their stem cells is shown on Fig. 1. The human promyelocytic leukemia cell line, designated HL-60, and the human monoblastic leukemia cell line, designated U937, are cells that differentiate to monocytes and/or granulocytes and are the models most frequently used to study the effects of $1,25(OH)_2D_3$ on hematopoietic differentiation. Exposure to $1,25(OH)_2D_3$ reduced the proliferation of these cells in liquid culture and decreased their clonal growth in soft agar. The expression of macrophage-related antigens and enzymes was increased and phagocytic activity was enhanced. The cells also gained the ability to degrade bone matrix [8,12–16]. These alterations were preceded by modulations in the expression of growth related protooncogenes characterized by a rapid decline in the levels of the mRNA for the protooncogene MYC [17,18], the transient expression of protooncogene FOS [18], and the sustained expression of the FMS protooncogene [19].

The $1,25(OH)_2D_3$ can inhibit growth and induce differentiation of myeloid leukemia cells in vitro. Myeloid leukemia cells cultured from nine patients showed significant differentiation when incubated with $10^{-7}M$ $1,25(OH)_2D_3$ for 6 days [20]. Lower concentrations of $1,25(OH)_2D_3$ did not

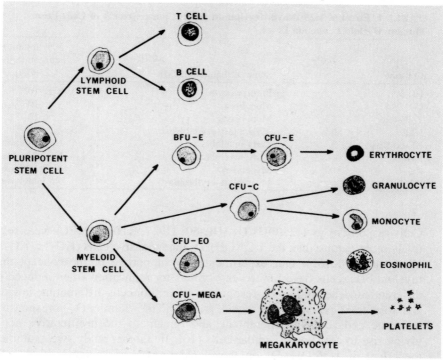

Fig. 1. Scheme of hematopoietic differentiation and proliferation. Abbreviations: BFU–E: erythrocyte burst forming unit; CFU–E: erythrocyte colony-forming unit; CFU–C: colony-forming unit in culture; CFU–EO: eosinophil colony-forming unit; CFU–MEGA: megakaryocyte colony-forming unit.

induce significant leukemic cell differentiation. Differentiation was assessed by cellular morphology, nitroblue tetrazolium reduction, and the ability to phagocytose yeast. The blast cells from more mature AML subtypes (M2,M4) showed greater ability to differentiate in the presence of $1,25(OH)_2D_3$ than an immature leukemic subtype (M1). In addition, $1,25(OH)_2D_3$ at concentrations of $10^{-7}M$, but not at lower concentrations, significantly inhibited growth of the leukemic cells in culture.

The effect of $1,25(OH)_2D_3$ on clonal proliferation of cells from eight myeloid leukemic lines is shown in Table I. The dose that inhibited 50% of the clonal growth (ED_{50}) of the responsive lines occurred at $1,25(OH)_2D_3$ concentrations between 2×10^{-8} and $2 \times 10^{-10}M$. These concentrations are comparable to the concentrations required for induction of differentiation in liquid culture [8]. Induction of differentiation in cell lines by $1,25(OH)_2D_3$ was always accompanied by inhibition of clonal growth of these cell lines.

TABLE I. Effect of 1,25-Dihydroxyvitamin D$_3$ on Clonal Growth of Cells From Human Myeloid Leukemia Lines

Cell line	Stage of maturation (M)	50% Inhibitory concentration 1,25(OH)$_2$D$_3$
HL-60	Promyelocyte	8×10^{-10}
U937	Monoblast	4×10^{-9}
THP-1	Monoblast	3×10^{-8}
HEL	Myeloblast–erythroblast	2×10^{-8}
HL-60 blast	Early myeloblast	No inhibition
KG-1a	Early myeloblast	No inhibition
KG-1	Myeloblast	No inhibition
K562	Myeloblast–erythroblast	No inhibition

Cells responsive to 1,25(OH)$_2$D$_3$ (HL-60, U937, THP-1, HEL) were relatively more mature than the 1,25(OH)$_2$D$_3$ unresponsive cells (KG-1a, KG-1, HL-60 blast, K562). Our experiments are supportive of the concept that myeloid blast cells have limited capabilities for replication when induced to differentiate. The vitamin D$_3$-responsive progenitor cells differentiate in vitro and lose their potential for clonal growth. The vitamin D$_3$-unresponsive leukemic cells do not differentiate and remain in the proliferative pool, giving rise to colonies of similar cells [16]. In another study, we examined the effect of 1,25(OH)$_2$D$_3$ on the clonal growth of leukemic blast cells harvested from either the peripheral blood or bone marrow of 14 patients with myeloid leukemia [16]. The ED$_{50}$ was about 5×10^{-7}M 1,25(OH)$_2$D$_3$ for leukemic blasts from 10 of the 14 patients. In contrast, 1,25(OH)$_2$D$_3$ stimulated the clonal proliferation of very immature blast cells from one AML patient by more than fourfold. Normal myeloid stem cells from 12 patients with myeloid leukemia in remission were neither inhibited nor stimulated by 1,25(OH)$_2$D$_3$.

The mechanism by which 1,25(OH)$_2$D$_3$ exerts its effects on myeloid cells is presently unclear. The HL-60 cells possess high affinity nuclear receptors for 1,25(OH)$_2$D$_3$ (vitamin D receptor, VDR) [8,12]. However, expression of these receptors is not sufficient to account for induction of differentiation. For example, the KG-1 cells have a comparable number of VDR to HL-60 but are resistant to the differentiation-inducing effects of 1,25(OH)$_2$D$_3$. Recently, cDNA clones encoding for chicken VDR, rat VDR, and human VDR have been isolated and the receptors have been characterized as a member of steroid–thyroid hormone receptor family on the basis of the DNA coding sequence [21–23]. The nucleotide sequences and the deduced amino acid sequences show that similarities exist among the VDR, the steroid hormone receptor, and the thyroid hormone receptor. Using Northern blot analysis, we

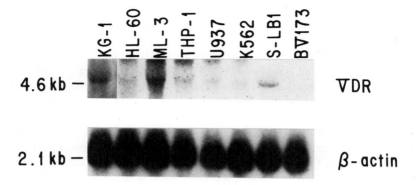

Fig. 2. Expression of 1,25(OH)$_2$D$_3$ receptor mRNA in human hematopoietic cell lines: KG-1 (myeloblasts), HL-60 (promyelocytes), ML-3 (early myeloblasts), THP-1, U937 (monoblasts), K562 (early myeloid/erythroid blast cells), S-LBI (HTLV-1 transformed T lymphocytes) and BV173 (B lymphocytes from a patient with lymphoid crisis of chronic myelogenous leukemia). Total RNA was extracted and analyzed by Northern blot technique and hybridized with [^{32}P]-labeled 1,25(OH)$_2$D$_3$ receptor cDNA. A single band could be detected at 4.6 kb consistent with 1,25(OH)$_2$D$_3$ receptor mRNA. The lower panel shows hybridization of the same RNAs with [^{32}P]-labeled β-actin cDNA (2.1 kb).

found that constitutive expression of VDR mRNA was detected in various kinds of hematopoietic cells including macrophage and activated T lymphocytes, as well as in various hematopoietic cell lines such as KG-1 (myeloblasts), HL-60 (promyelocytes), ML-3 (early myelomonoblasts), U937, THP-1 (monoblasts), K562 (erythroid blast cells), and S-LBI (HTLV-1 transformed T lymphocytes) [24] (Fig. 2). Furthermore, levels of expression of VDR mRNA were not modulated by exposure to ligand [i.e., 1,25(OH)$_2$D$_3$] and steady-state levels of VDR mRNA were not affected by terminal differentiation of HL-60 towards granulocytes or macrophages [24]. Structural similarities between 1,25(OH)$_2$D$_3$ and the ''classical'' steroid hormones suggest that 1,25(OH)$_2$D$_3$ might passively enter the nuclear compartment of cells and complex with its specific receptor bound to specific regions of DNA. Transcription of the gene, where binding occurs, might then be altered. Why 1,25(OH)$_2$D$_3$ preferentially inhibits in vitro the proliferation of leukemic, but not normal human myeloid stem cells is not clear. Differences in receptor number or affinity, or the activation of different genes and metabolic pathways may account for this differential effect.

EFFECTS OF 1,25(OH)$_2$D$_3$ ON LYMPHOCYTES

Receptors for 1,25(OH)$_2$D$_3$ are expressed in activated, proliferating human B and T lymphocytes, but these receptors cannot be detected in quiescent lymphocytes [25]. The VDRs are also found in cells from transformed lymphocyte lines. Research in the past 3 years has revealed a large spectrum of effects of $1,25(OH)_2D_3$ on lymphocytes.

The hormone inhibited the synthesis of DNA and the proliferation of lectin-activated human lymphocytes [26]. These effects were probably mediated through a repression of interleukin-2 production [26]. This repression occurred at the mRNA level [27], although $1,25(OH)_2D_3$ had no influence on the number of interleukin-2 receptors. The hormone also suppressed the production by lectin-activated lymphocytes of two other immunologically active lymphokines: granulocyte–macrophage colony-stimulating factor and gamma-interferon [28,29]. This could be demonstrated at both the mRNA and protein levels and was independent of DNA synthesis and interleukin-2 production rates. The $1,25(OH)_2D_3$-induced inhibition of the synthesis of granulocyte–macrophage colony-stimulating factor was at a posttranscriptional level [29]. Other studies have shown that $1,25(OH)_2D_3$ has inhibitory effects on the synthesis of immunoglobulins by B lymphocytes; these effects are either exerted directly on B lymphocytes [30] or mediated indirectly by T helper-cell activity [31]. The relevance of these new findings to osteoporosis is not clear; studies have shown that the ratio of helper to suppressor cells is increased in patients with spinal fracture and that administration of $1\alpha(OH)D_3$ corrects this irregularity [32].

CLINICAL STUDY OF $1,25(OH)_2D_3$ AND DEVELOPMENT OF NOVEL VITAMIN D_3 COMPOUNDS

We initiated a trial of administering $1,25(OH)_2D_3$ to patients with myelodysplastic syndromes (MDS) because of the ability of the vitamin D_3 metabolite to induce differentiation and to inhibit the clonal proliferation of some human acute myelogenous leukemia cells. Studies have also shown that administration of $1\alpha(OH)D_3$ significantly prolonged the life of mice injected with the M1 transplantable murine leukemia cells [33]. We chose to study myelodysplastic patients because the tempo of their disease allows scrutiny of therapeutic maneuvers. Patients with MDS usually have their leukemic clone established; they have ineffective hematopoiesis, almost always with anemia and frequently thrombocytopenia, leukopenia, and often an increased number of marrow blast cells. Eighteen patients with MDS were given weekly escalating doses (0.5 µg) of $1,25(OH)_2D_3$ up to 2 µg/day for a median duration of 12 weeks of therapy [20]. Eight patients experienced an improvement in at least one hematologic parameter for more than 4 weeks. In spite of this, no patient had improvement in their peripheral blood counts or bone marrow blast counts by the end of the study (≥ 12 weeks). Seven of the patients developed acute leukemia during the trial. The major dose-limiting toxicity was hypercalcemia, which developed in nine patients. Perhaps this trial failed to show a significant therapeutic effect because of the dose-limiting toxicity of $1,25(OH)_2D_3$. Serum concentrations of $1,25(OH)_2D_3$ reached $2 \times 10^{-10}M$ with the administration of 2 μg/day. For comparison, concentrations of between 5×10^{-9} and $5 \times 10^{-8}M$ $1,25(OH)_2D_3$ are required to induce significant differentiation of myeloid leukemia blasts in vitro.

Attempts are currently being directed toward the identification of chemically modified vitamin D_3 analogs that induce hematopoietic cell differentiation without inducing hypercalcemia. These might be medically useful compounds for selected patients with MDS and acute leukemia [34–37].

Seven new analogs of $1,25(OH)_2D_3$ were discovered to be either equivalent or more potent than $1,25(OH)_2D_3$ as assessed by (1) inhibition of clonal proliferation of HL-60, EM-2, U937, and patients' myeloid leukemic cells; and (2) induction of differentiation of HL-60 promyelocytes. Furthermore, these analogs stimulated clonal growth of normal human myeloid stem cells. The most potent analog, 1,25-dihydroxy-16ene-23yne-vitamin D_3 was about fourfold more potent than $1,25(OH)_2D_3$. This analog decreased both clonal growth and expression of c-myc RNA in HL-60 cells by 50% within 10 hr of exposure. Effects on calcium metabolism of the novel analogs in vivo was assessed by intestinal calcium absorption (ICA) and bone calcium mobilization (BCM). Each of the analogs mediated markedly less (10- to 200-fold) ICA and BCM as compared with $1,25(OH)_2D_3$. To gain insight into the possible mechanism of action of these new analogs, receptor binding studies with $1,25(OH)_2$-16ene-23yne-D_3 showed that it competed only about 60% as effectively as $1,25(OH)_2D_3$ for $1,25(OH)_2D_3$ receptors present in HL-60 cells and 98% as effective as $1,25(OH)_2D_3$ for receptors present in chick intestinal cells [37].

The therapeutic potential of $1,25(OH)_2$-16ene-23yne-D_3 was explored by developing and using three leukemia models: (1) Injection of 2.5×10^5 myeloid leukemic cells (WEHI–3BD$^+$) into syngeneic BALB/c mice resulted in leukemic death of all control mice who received injection of only diluent by day 26. Mice who received the same number of leukemic cells and also received $1,25(OH)_2D_3$ (0.1 μg every other day [q.o.d.], intraperitonealy [I.P.]) had nearly an identical survival curve. Those who received the leukemic cells and $1,25(OH)_2$-16ene-23yne-D_3 (1.6 μg q.o.d., I.P.) had a significantly (P = 0.003) longer survival, with the last mouse dying of leukemia on day 50. (2) Injection of 60% fewer leukemic cells (1×10^5) into syngeneic BALB/c mice resulted in 86% mortality rate from leukemia at 51 days. In contrast, experimental mice who received the same number of leukemic cells and $1,25(OH)_2$-16ene-23yne-D_3 (0.8 μg q.o.d.) had a significantly (P = 0.0006) longer survival than controls; only 53% of the mice were dead by day 100. (3) After injection of 1.5×10^4 leukemic cells, only 13% of syngeneic BALB/c mice were free of disease at day 180. In contrast, 43% of mice who received leukemic cells and $1,25(OH)_2$-16ene-23yne-D_3 (1.6 μg q.o.d.) were still free of disease at day 180 [38]. In summary, these novel vitamin D_3 analogs are more potent than physiologic $1,25(OH)_2D_3$ in inducing differentiation and inhibiting proliferation of leukemic cells. Moreover, these compounds appear to have the potential to be markedly less toxic as measured by the development of hypercalcemia. For example, about 10-fold more $1,25(OH)_2$-16ene-23yne-D_3 is required to produce hypercalcemia as compared to $1,25(OH)_2D_3$. These novel vitamin D_3 analogs may prove superior to $1,25(OH)_2D_3$ in a number of clinical situations including MDS and acute leukemia. In addition, they will provide a tool to dissect the mechanism of action of vitamin D_3 seco-steroids in promoting cellular differentiation.

MACROPHAGES AND SYNTHESIS OF $1,25(OH)_2D_3$

Several lines of evidence suggest that cells, other than kidney cells, are capable of synthesis of $1,25(OH)_2D_3$. Normal circulating levels of $1,25(OH)_2D_3$ are in the range of 30–50 pg/ml. Although these serum concentrations markedly decrease in nephrectomized patients, some investigators reported persistent serum $1,25(OH)_2D_3$ levels in the range of 5–10 pg/ml [39]. We find that 20–30% of patients with sarcoidosis have hypercalcemia and elevated serum levels of $1,25(OH)_2D_3$. One study demonstrated increased serum $1,25(OH)_2D_3$ in a nephrectomized patient with sarcoidosis [40]. These studies provide support for the hypothesis that cells, other than cells from the kidney, can produce $1,25(OH)_2D_3$. Likewise, Adams et al. [41] reported that pulmonary alveolar macrophages harvested from patients with sarcoidosis are capable of constitutively converting the substrate [^{3}H]-$25(OH)D_3$ to [^{3}H]-$1,25(OH)_2D_3$ [41].

Patients with sarcoidosis have activated T lymphocytes that secrete large amounts of gamma interferon (gamma-IFN). A reasonable hypothesis is that perhaps gamma-IFN might stimulate normal human macrophages to produce $1,25(OH)_2D_3$. We found that gamma-IFN markedly enhanced the ability of normal human macrophages to synthesize a vitamin D_3 metabolite that migrates on HPLC in exact identity with authentic, chemically synthesized $1,25(OH)_2D_3$ [10]. We rechromatographed the putative $1,25(OH)_2D_3$ using three other high-performance liquid chromatography (HPLC) elution systems. In each system the [^{3}H]-metabolite ran in exact identity with $1,25(OH)_2D_3$.

The $1,25(OH)_2D_3$-like material produced by the macrophage was purified to homogeneity and was identified as $1,25(OH)_2D_3$ by (1) characteristic affinity for the chicken intestinal $1,25(OH)_2D_3$ receptor [42]; (2) identical biological activity with that of chemically synthesized $1,25(OH)_2D_3$ in vivo (intestinal calcium absorption and bone calcium mobilization in rachitic chickens) [43]; and (3) mass spectroscopy showing the typical spectral pattern of $1,25(OH)_2D_3$ [42].

The ability of normal human pulmonary alveolar macrophages to synthesize putative $1,25(OH)_2D_3$ has been examined in cells obtained from more than 20 normal volunteers. Although results varied quantitatively from patient to patient, we found that gamma-IFN was able to enhance the synthesis of $1,25(OH)_2D_3$ between 10- and 200-fold as compared to macrophages not exposed to the lymphokine. Dose-response studies showed that the ability of the macrophages to synthesize $1,25(OH)_2D_3$ increased with exposure of the cells to increasing concentrations of gamma-IFN with the earliest effects being noted at 200 units/ml of gamma-IFN. Maximally stimulated macrophages synthesized about 10–50 pmol of $1,25(OH)_2D_3/10^6$ cells in several hours. Time-response studies showed that maximal stimulation occurred within 24 hr of exposure of the macrophages to gamma-IFN (500 u/ml); stimulation of the macrophages was evident for at least 6 days. Inactivated gamma-IFN did not stimulate macrophages to synthesize $1,25(OH)_2D_3$. These studies suggest that gamma-IFN can stimulate synthesis of $1,25(OH)_2D_3$ by macrophages. Further studies showed that lipopolysaccharide was also a potent stimulator of the synthesis of $1,25(OH)_2D_3$ by human macrophages [43]. Activation of macrophages is probably necessary for $1,25(OH)_2D_3$ production by macrophages.

COMMUNICATION BETWEEN MACROPHAGES AND T LYMPHOCYTES

Activated macrophages and lymphocytes may communicate by using a vitamin D_3 paracrine system. For example, after exposure to microorganisms, macrophages synthesize IL-1 and present antigens of the microbes to T lymphocytes. The combination of IL-1 and antigen presentation leads to activation of T lymphocytes. These activated T lymphocytes synthesize IL-2 and a variety of cytokines including gamma-IFN and GM–CSF. Gamma-IFN will further activate the macrophages to perform their microbicidal activities more efficiently. Gamma-IFN will also stimulate the local production of $1,25(OH)_2D_3$ by these macrophages. In low concentrations, this $1,25(OH)_2D_3$ may enhance the number of macrophages by stimulating preferential differentiation of the myeloid stem cell towards macrophages and may also act as a negative regulatory signal for adjacent lymphocytes producing a down-modulation of the immune response [9,26,28,30,31,44].

REFERENCES

1. Haussler MR, McCain TA (1977): Basic and clinical concepts related to vitamin D metabolism and action. N Engl J Med 297:974–83 and 1041–1050.
2. DeLuca HF, Schnoes HK (1983): Vitamin D: Recent advances. Annu Rev Biochem 52:411–439.
3. Norman AW, Roth J, Orci L (1982): The vitamin D endocrine system: Steroid metabolism hormone receptors, and biological response (calcium binding proteins). Endocr Rev 3: 331–336.
4. McCarthy DJ, Hibbin JF, San Miguel JF, Freake HC, Rodriguez B, Andrews C, Pining A, Catovsky D, Goldman JM (1984): The effect of vitamin D_3 metabolites on normal and leukemic bone marrow cells in vitro. Int J Cell Cloning 2:227–242.
5. Koeffler HP, Armatruda T, Ikekawa N, Kobayashi Y, DeLuca HF (1984): Induction of macrophage differentiation of human normal and leukemic myeloid stem cells by 1,25-dihydroxyvitamin D_3 and its fluorinated analogues. Cancer Res 44:5624–5628.
6. Tanaka H, Abe E, Miyaura C, Kuribayashi T, Konno K, Nishii Y, Suda T (1982): 1 alpha, 25-dihydroxycholecalciferol and a human myeloid leukemic cell line (HL-60). The presence of a cytosol receptor and induction of differentiation. Biochem J 204:713–719.
7. Olsson J, Gulberg U, Ivbed J, Nilsson K (1983): Induction of differentiation of the human histiocytic lymphoma cell line u937 by 1 alpha, 25-dihydroxycholecalciferol. Cancer Res 43:5862–5867.
8. Mangelsdorf DJ, Koeffler HP, Donaldson CA, Pike JW, Haussler MR (1984): 1,25-Dihydroxyvitamin D_3-induced differentiation in a human promyelocytic leukemia cell line (HL-60). Receptor-mediated maturation to macrophage-like cells. J Cell Biol 98:391–398.
9. Rigby WFC, Shen L, Ball ED, Juyre PM, Fanger FW (1984): Differentiation of a human monocytic cell line by 1,25-dihydroxyvitamin D_3 (calcitriol): a morphologic, phenotypic, and functional analysis. Blood 64:1110–1115.
10. Koeffler HP, Reichel H, Bishop JE, Norman AW (1985): Gamma-interferon stimulates production of 1,25-dihydroxyvitamin D_3 by normal human macrophage. Biochem Biophys Res Commun 127:596–603.
11. Abe E, Miyaura C, Sakagami H, Takeda M, Konno K, Yamazaki T, Yoshiki S, Suda T (1981): Differentiation of mouse myeloid leukemia cells induced by $1\alpha,25$-dihydroxyvitamin D_3. Proc Natl Acad Sci USA 78:4990–4994.
12. Bar-Shavit Z, Teitelbaum SL, Reitsma P, Hall A, Pegg LE, Trial J, Kahn AJ (1983): Monocytic differentiation and bone resorption by 1,25-dihydroxyvitamin D_3. Proc Natl Acad Sci USA 80:5907–5911.
13. McCarthy DM, San Miguel TF, Freake HC (1983): 1,25-Dihydroxyvitamin D_3 inhibits proliferation of human promyelocytic leukaemia (HL-60) cells and induces monocyte-macrophage differentiation of HL-60 and normal human bone marrow cells. Leuk Res 7: 51–55.
14. Dodd RC, Cohen MS, Newman SL, Gray TK (1983): Vitamin D metabolites change the phenotype of monoblastic U937 cells. Proc Natl Acad Sci USA 80:7538–7541.
15. Amento EP, Bhalla AK, Kurnick JT, Kradin RL, Clemens TL, Holick MF, Holick SA, Krane SH (1984): $1\alpha,25$-Dihydroxyvitamin D_3 induces maturation of the human monocyte cell line U937, and, in association with a factor from human T lymphocytes, augments production of the monokine mononuclear cell factor. J Clin Invest 73:731–739.
16. Munker R, Norman AW, Koeffler HP (1986): Vitamin D compounds. Effect on clonal proliferation and differentiation of human myeloid cells. J Clin Invest 78:424–430.
17. Simpson RU, Hsu T, Begley DA, Mitchell BS, Alizadeh BN (1987): Transcriptional

regulation of the c-myc protooncogene by 1,25-dihydroxyvitamin D_3 in HL-60 promyelocytic leukemia cells. J Biol Chem 262:4104–4108.

18. Brelvi ZS, Studzinski GP (1986): Changes in the expression of oncogenes encoding nuclear phosphoproteins but not c-Ha-ras have a relationship to monocytic differentiation of HL-60 cells. J Cell Biol 102:2234–2243.

19. Scariban E, Mitchell T, Kufe D (1985): Expression of the c-fms proto-oncogene during human monocytic differentiation. Nature 316:64–66.

20. Koeffler HP, Hirji K, Itri L (1985): 1,25-Dihydroxyvitamin D_3: In vivo and in vitro effects on human preleukemic and leukemic cells. Cancer Treatment Rep 69:1399–1406.

21. McDonnell DP, Mangelsdorf DJ, Pike JW, Haussler MR, O'Malley BW (1987): Molecular cloning of complementary DNA encoding the avian receptor for vitamin D. Science 235:1214–1217.

22. Burmester JK, Wiese RJ, Malda N, DeLuca HF (1988): Structure and regulation of the rat 1,25-dihydroxyvitamin D_3 receptor. Proc Natl Acad Sci USA 85:9499–9502.

23. Baker AR, McDonnel DP, Hughes M, Crisp TM, Mangelsdorf DJ, Haussler MR, Pike JW, Shine J, O'Malley BW (1988): Cloning and expression of full-length cDNA encoding human vitamin D receptor. Proc Natl Acad Sci USA 85:3294–3298.

24. Kizaki M, Lin CW, Karmaker A, Koeffler HP (1990): 1,25-Dihydroxyvitamin D_3 receptor RNA: expression in hematopoietic cells (submitted).

25. Provvedini DM, Tsoukas CD, Deftos LJ, Manolagas SC (1983): 1,25-Dihydroxyvitamin D_3 receptors in human leukocytes. Science 221:1181–1183.

26. Tsoukas CD, Provvedini DM, Manolagas SC (1984): 1,25-Dihydroxyvitamin D_3: A novel immunoregulatory hormone. Science 224:1438–1440.

27. Rigby WFC, Denome S, Fanger FW (1987): Regulation of lymphokine production and human T lymphocyte activation by 1,25-dihydroxyvitamin D_3. Specific inhibition at the level of messenger RNA. J Clin Invest 79:1659–1664.

28. Reichel H, Koeffler HP, Tobler A, Norman AW (1987): 1α-25-Dihydroxyvitamin D_3 inhibits interferon-gamma synthesis by normal human peripheral blood lymphocytes. Proc Natl Acad Sci USA 1987:3385–3389.

29. Tobler A, Miller CW, Norman AW, Koeffler HP (1988): 1,25-dihydroxyvitamin D_3 modulates the expression of a lymphokine (granulocyte-macrophage colony-stimulating factor) postranscriptionally. J Clin Invest 81:1819–1823.

30. Iho S, Takahashi T, Kura F, Sugiyama H, Hoshino T (1986): The effect of 1,25-dihydroxyvitamin D_3 on in vitro immunoglobulin production in human B cells. J Immunol 236:4427–4431.

31. Lemire JM, Adams JS, Kermani-Arab V, Bakke AC, Sakai R, Jordan SC (1984): 1,25-Dihydroxyvitamin D_3 suppresses human T helper/inducer lymphocyte activity in vitro. J Immunol 134:3032–3035.

32. Fujita T, Matsui T, Nakao Y, Watanabe S (1984): T lymphocyte subsets in osteoporosis. Effect of 1-alpha hydroxyvitamin D_3. Mineral Electr Metab 10:375–378.

33. Honma Y, Hozumi M, Abe E, Konnao K, Fukushima M, Hata S, Nishii Y, DeLuca H, Suda T (1983): 1α,25-Dihydroxyvitamin D_3 and 1α-hydroxyvitamin D_3 prolong survival time of mice inoculated with myeloid leukemia cells. Proc Natl Acad Sci USA 80: 201–204.

34. Ostrem VK, Tanaka Y, Prahl J, DeLuca HF, Ikekawa N (1987): 24- and 26-Homo-1,25-dihydroxyvitamin D_3: preferential activity in inducing differentiation of huma leukemic cells HL-60 in vitro. Proc Natl Acad Sci USA 84:2610–2614.

35. Inaba M, Okumo S, Nishizawa Y, Yukioka K, Otani S, Yuasa IM, Morisawa S, DeLuca HF, Morii H (1987): Biological activity of fluorinated vitamin D analogs at C-26 and C-27 on human promyelocytic leukemia cells, HL-60. Arch Biochem Biophys 258:421–425.

36. Abe J, Morikawa M, Miyamoto K, Kaiho S, Fukushima M, Miyaura C, Abe E, Suda T, Nishii Y (1987): Synthetic analogues of vitamin D_3 with an oxygen atom in the side chain skeleton. FEBS Lett 226:58–62.

37. Zhou HY, Norman AW, Lubbert M, Collins ED, Uskokovic MR, Koeffler HP (1989): Novel vitamin D analogs that modulate leukemic cell growth and differentiation with little effect on either intestinal calcium absorption or bone metabolization. Blood 74:82–93.

38. Zhou JY, Norman AW, Chen DL, Uskokovic M, Koeffler HP (1990): 1,25(OH)$_2$-16ene-23yne-vitamin D_3 prolongs survival time of leukemic mice. Proc Natl Acad Sci USA 87:3929–3932.

39. Lambert PW, Stern PH, Avioli RC, Brackett NC, Turner RT, Green A, Irene YF, Bell NH (1982): Evidence for extrarenal production of 1α-25-dihydroxyvitamin D in man. J Clin Invest 69:722–725.

40. Barbour GL, Coburn JW, Slatopolsky E, Norman AW, Horst RL (1981): Hypercalcemia in an anephric patient with sarcoidosis: Evidence for extrarenal generation of 1,25-dihydroxyvitamin D. N Engl J Med 305:440–448.

41. Adams JS, Sharma OP, Gacad MA, Singer FR (1983): Metabolism of 25-hydroxyvitamin D_3 by cultured pulmonary alveolar macrophage in sarcoidosis. J Clin Invest 72:1856–1860.

42. Reichel H, Koeffler HP, Norman AW (1987): Synthesis *in vitro* of 1,25-dihydroxyvitamin D_3 and 24,25-dihydroxyvitamin D_3 by interferon-gamma stimulated normal human bone marrow and alveolar macrophage. J Biol Chem 262:10931–10937.

43. Reichel H, Koeffler HP, Bishop JE, Norman AW (1987): 25-Hydroxyvitamin D_3 metabolism by lipopolysaccharide-stimulated normal human macrophage. J Clin Endocrinol Metab 64:1–9.

44. Tobler A, Gasson J, Reichel H, Norman AW, Koeffler HP (1987): Granulocyte-macrophage colony-stimulating factor. Sensitive and receptor-mediated regulation by 1,25-dihydroxyvitamin D_3 in normal human peripheral blood lymphocytes. J Clin Invest 79:1700–1705.

Vitamins and Cancer Prevention, pages 103–110
© 1991 Wiley-Liss, Inc.

8 | Coenzyme Q_{10} Deficiency in Cancer Patients: Potential for Immunotherapy With Coenzyme Q_{10}?

Karl Folkers
John Ellis
Ovid Yang
Hiroo Tamagawa

Yoshio Nara
Kimiyo Nara
Chun-qu Ye
Zongxuan Shen

INTRODUCTION

Coenzyme Q_{10} (CoQ_{10}), a lipid-soluble coenzyme, is one of a family of compounds known as ubiquinones. These compounds, which are structurally similar, differing only in the length of the isoprenoid side chain (Fig. 1) are found in animals, plants, and microorganisms. Coenzyme Q_{10}, which is found in mitochondria of animals, is thought to function as a transporter of

Institute for Biomedical Research, University of Texas at Austin, Austin, TX 78712 (K.F., H.T., Y.N., K.N., C-q.Y., Z.S.); Titus County Memorial Hospital, Mt. Pleasant, Texas, 75455 (J.E., O.Y.)

electrons from organic substrates to oxygen in the mitochondrial respiratory chain. It functions by reversible addition of two electrons.

It is presently believed that CoQ_{10} is synthesized widely within the human body. Tyrosine is the precursor for the quinone nucleus of CoQ_{10}, and the multistep biosynthetic conversion of tyrosine to CoQ_{10} is a biochemical mechanism requiring several nutrients, including vitamins, cofactors, and trace elements [1]. Any single deficiency or multiple deficiencies of these nutrients can cause reduced cellular levels of CoQ_{10}; in cancer patients varied and diverse nutritional deficiencies may exist.

Over the past three decades of working with animal models, we have demonstrated both a hematological and an immunological role for CoQ_{10}. The hematological activities of the CoQ group in animal models appear to

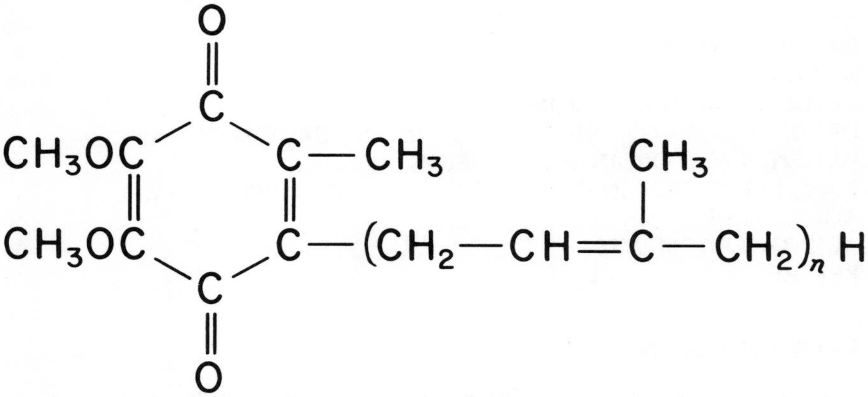

Fig. 1. Structure of Coenzyme Q. $n = 10$ for Coenzyme Q_{10}.

involve two modes of action: (1) bioenergetic activities in mitochondria and (2) antioxidant activities. Coenzyme Q_{10} may have a secondary role that is protective against peroxidation. In contrast, the immunological activity of CoQ_{10}, including its effect on IgG biosynthesis, is based principally, perhaps exclusively, upon its bioenergetic role.

We would like to review the importance of the role of CoQ_{10} in blood cell function and in immunological activity, prior to describing a potentially exciting observation of CoQ_{10} deficiency in cancer patients.

HEMATOLOGICAL ACTIVITY OF COENZYME Q

Between 1962 and 1967, we described the hematological activity of members of the CoQ group in a series of both animal and human studies. Experimental and nutritional anemia in monkeys responded to treatment with the 6-chromanol of hexahydrocoenzyme Q_4 (H_6CoQ_4) [2]. Similarly, H_6CoQ_4 was also observed to have hematopoietic activity in the monkey [3, 4]. These observations were followed by elucidation of the hematological activity of CoQ_{10} in the monkey [5].

In nutritionally deficient children, macrocytic anemia responded to treatment with the 6-chromanol of CoQ_4 [6, 7]. Hexahydrocoenzyme Q_4 and particularly CoQ_{10} were also observed to exert hematopoietic activity in anemic children. This report suggested potential clinical significance because these studies involved the effect of CoQ_{10} on human tissues. This enhancement of hematopoietic activity of CoQ_{10} was also observed in other animal species, including chickens and turkeys; H_6CoQ_4 exhibited a similar effect [8]. Subsequent studies have evaluated the hematological activities of several CoQ species in rabbits, chickens, turkeys, monkeys, and children [9].

The mechanisms underlying these hematological activities are understood to be based upon the antioxidant activities of the 6-chromanols of members of the CoQ group, although this antioxidant activity may be principally expressed through protection of CoQ_{10}. In contrast, CoQ_{10} appears to stimulate hematopoiesis based primarily upon its bioenergetic role in mitochondria. This indispensable mitochondrial activity may be protected by antioxidants such as vitamin E.

IMMUNOLOGICAL ACTIVITY OF COENZYME Q

Further studies by our group and others, have described a beneficial effect of CoQ_{10} on immunological activity. Emulsions of CoQ_6 and CoQ_{10} were found to increase phagocytic activity in rats [10]. Casey and Bliznakov [11] subsequently observed that CoQ_{10} was more effective than CoQ_6 or H_6CoQ_4 in increasing the rate of phagocytosis in rats, while coenzyme Q_0 (CoQ_0), $H_{20}CoQ_{10}$, the 6-chromanols of CoQ and vitamin E were ineffective. These observations gave clues to the understanding of the mechanism of this effect. Administration of CoQ_{10} was observed to reduce the incidence of chemically induced tumors (from dibenzpyrene) in mice, and to increase survival rates [12]. Administration of CoQ_{10} also increased survival rates of mice that had been infected with the Friend leukemia virus. It was concluded that CoQ_{10} administration enhanced host defense systems essential for protection against carcinogens and viruses. Later studies in mice revealed that Friend leukemia virus infection resulted in deficiency of a CoQ_{10}–enzyme [13]. Coenzyme Q_{10} has also been proposed as a potential agent protecting against senescence [14]. Deficiency of a CoQ_{10}–enzyme appears to increase in the thymus of mice as their age increases, while the weight of the thymus gland decreases [15]. Some human studies have been carried out; clinical administration of CoQ_{10} increased IgG levels in eight patients, three of whom had cancer, four had cardiovascular disease, and one had diabetes [16].

Thus, although antioxidants, vitamin E, and the 6-chromanols of CoQ do not significantly stimulate immunological activity, CoQ_{10} appears to enhance immunological activity, possibly through stimulation of the host defense system. Underlying such a stimulation may be a CoQ_{10}-induced stimulation of bioenergetic functions in mitochondria. If this stimulation of bioenergetic activity by CoQ_{10} in mitochondria is generalized and if cancer patients are deficient in CoQ_{10}, there is the potential for immunotherapy by CoQ_{10} in diverse cancer patients.

METHODS

Whole blood specimens of 22 cancer patients (9 females and 13 males) were drawn on the occasion of the first diagnosis, before pathological identification of the cancer, and prior to initiation of chemotherapy or radiation therapy. Subsequent cancer pathology revealed carcinomas of the thyroid, esophagus, colon, breast, lung, skin and neck, and uterus. Coenzyme Q_{10} levels in whole blood were measured by high-performance liquid chromatography (HPLC) [17]. Blood levels of CoQ_{10} of these cancer patients are shown in Table I. Statistical analyses of these blood levels of CoQ_{10} in comparison with control data without regard to the age of the subjects are shown in Table II. Comparison of the data from the cancer patients with age-matched controls are shown in Tables III and IV.

RESULTS AND DISCUSSION

In the 22 patients we studied, blood levels of CoQ_{10} ranged from 0.32 to 1.35 μg/ml (Table I). We compared these data with blood levels of control subjects. The word, "control" rather than "normal" is used to designate these subjects to avoid the implication that "normal" means "healthy."

TABLE I. Blood Level of Coenzyme Q₁₀ of Newly Diagnosed and Untreated Cancer Patients

Patient	Age	Sex	Blood level (μg/ml)
1	33	F	0.49
2	44	F	0.54
3	58	M	1.09
4	62	F	0.63
5	63	F	1.01
6	65	F	0.60
7	69	M	1.35
8	69	M	1.03
9	70	M	0.49
10	71	M	0.99
11	71	M	0.32
12	72	F	0.91
13	75	F	0.51
14	76	M	0.75
15	76	M	0.78
16	76	F	0.48
17	78	M	0.47
18	80	M	0.72
19	81	F	0.52
20	83	M	0.61
21	85	F	0.34
22	90	M	0.60

TABLE II. Statistical Analyses of CoQ_{10} Levels

Comparison of the Whole Groups

CoQ_{10} (μg/ml)	Control subjects (N = 215)	Cancer patients (N = 22)	X2	p Value
<0.65	61	13	8.770	$p < 0.005$
<0.60	36	9	7.576	$p < 0.005$
<0.55	24	9	14.734	$p < 0.005$
<0.50	12	6	13.380	$p < 0.005$
<0.40	2	2	8.010	$p < 0.005$
<0.35	0	2	19.712	$p < 0.005$

Although in most subjects this may be true, we sought to avoid this semantic pitfall. Thus, these subjects were available and cooperated in allowing blood specimens to be drawn and had no overt deficiency or disease, but may have had deficiency or disease that was not overt. Also, the control subjects did not report taking vitamin supplements; such supplemental vitamins might facilitate cellular CoQ_{10} biosynthesis.

TABLE III. Statistical Analyses of CoQ_{10} Levels

Comparison of Individuals above 32 Years

CoQ_{10} (μg/ml)	Control subjects (N = 38)	Cancer patients (N = 22)	X2	p Value
<0.70	8	13	8.862	p < 0.005
<0.65	7	13	10.371	p < 0.005
<0.60	5	9	5.998	p < 0.005
<0.55	3	9	9.492	p < 0.005
<0.50	1	6	8.209	p < 0.005

TABLE IV. Statistical Analyses of CoQ_{10} Levels

Comparison of Individuals above 39 Years

CoQ_{10} (μg/ml)	Control subjects (N = 18)	Cancer patients (N = 22)	X2	p Value
<0.70	4	12	4.885	p < 0.05
<0.60	3	12	6.709	p < 0.01
<0.55	0	5	4.916	p < 0.05

In a recent study, we measured CoQ_{10} in blood from control subjects without overt deficiency or disease; CoQ_{10} levels ranged from 0.3 to 1.6 μg/ml (mean value, 0.79 ± 0.22 μg/ml, n = 234) [18]. Thus, an initial inspection of the data suggested that the range of blood CoQ_{10} was the same for the 22 cancer patients in the present study and 234 control subjects in this previous study from our group. In addition to these data, we have subsequently measured CoQ_{10} in 215 control subjects stratified according to age. These blood CoQ_{10} levels were used in the present statistical analyses of Tables II–IV.

Serum CoQ_{10} is probably derived from CoQ_{10} released during cellular turnover in the tissues of the entire body. This serum level of CoQ_{10} is substantially greater than that in the white cell population. Therefore, low blood levels of CoQ_{10} may reflect a deficiency in body tissues, while high blood levels may or may not reflect a deficiency.

If the serum level of CoQ_{10} is representative of cellular turnover in the entire body, and if whole blood levels may not correlate with functional organ levels of CoQ_{10}, it may not be particularly meaningful to compare mean levels of CoQ_{10} in cancer patients and in control subjects. However, the incidence of low levels of CoQ_{10} in the blood of cancer patients can be meaningful in comparison with the incidence of low blood levels of control subjects.

INCIDENCE OF COQ$_{10}$ DEFICIENCIES IN THE GROUPS OF CANCER PATIENTS AND ORDINARY SUBJECTS

We stratified both the cancer patients and the control subjects by their levels of CoQ$_{10}$. In Table II, we compared the data on CoQ$_{10}$ blood levels for the 22 cancer patients with that from those individuals among the 215 control subjects who had blood levels of CoQ$_{10}$ between 0 and 0.65 , 0.60, 0.55, 0.50, 0.40, and 0.35 µg/ml. Within each of these ranges of CoQ$_{10}$ levels, the incidence of a CoQ$_{10}$ deficiency in the blood of the cancer patients was greater than ($p < 0.005$) was the incidence of a CoQ$_{10}$ deficiency in the control subjects. For example, 59% of the 22 cancer patients had blood levels of CoQ$_{10}$ less than 0.65 µg/ml ($p < 0.005$); in contrast, 28% of the control subjects exhibited levels this low.

CoQ$_{10}$ DEFICIENCY IN CANCER PATIENTS AS BASED ON TWO AGE LEVELS

We then attempted to remove possible age-related changes in CoQ$_{10}$ levels. The minimum age of the cancer patients was 33 years. In Table III, we compared blood CoQ$_{10}$ levels of cancer patients with those of control subjects who were over 32 years of age. We found that 13 out of 22 cancer patients (59%) had blood levels below 0.7 µg/ml. Of the 215 control subjects, 38 were over 32 years in age and 8 of those 38 subjects (21%) had CoQ$_{10}$ blood levels below 0.7 µg/ml. Therefore, the incidence of low blood CoQ$_{10}$ levels was higher ($p < 0.005$) in the cancer patients than in approximately age-matched control subjects. None of the 38 control subjects had blood levels of CoQ$_{10}$ below 0.45 µg/ml, but 6/22 (27%) cancer patients had levels below 0.45 µg/ml.

In Table IV, blood levels of CoQ$_{10}$ for control subjects and cancer patients are compared on the basis of the "older individuals," that is, above 39 years. Of the 215 control subjects, 18 were 39 years or older and 18 of the 22 cancer patients were older than 39 years. None of the 18 control subjects had CoQ$_{10}$ blood levels below 0.5 µg/ml, but 5 of the 18 cancer patients (27%) had blood levels below 0.5 µg/ml ($p < 0.05$).

ACKNOWLEDGMENTS

Appreciation is expressed to the Robert A. Welch Foundation of Houston, Texas.

REFERENCES

1. Friedrich W (1988): "Vitamins." New York: Walter de Gruyter, pp 590–591.
2. Dinning JS, Fitch CD, Shunk CH, Folkers K (1962): J Am Chem Soc 84: 2007–2008.

3. Farley TM, Scholler J, Smith JL, Folkers K, Fitch A (1967): Arch Biochem Biophys 121, 625–632.

4. Ludwig FC, Elashoff RM, Smith JL, Scholler J, Farley TM, Folkers K (1967): Scand J Haematol 4: 292–300.

5. Fitch CD, Dinning JS, Porter FS, Folkers K, Moore HW, Smith JL (1964): Arch Biochem Biophys 112: 488–493.

6. Dinning JS, Majaj AS, Assmam SA, Darby WJ, Skunk CH, Folkers K (1963): Am J Clin Nutr 13: 169–172.

7. Majaj AS, Dinning JS, Folkers K (1963) Abstract from the 9th Congress of the European Society of Hematology, Lisbon, August 26–31, 1963.

8. Larsen M, Couch JR, Enzmann F, Boler L, Mustafa H, Folkers K (1969): Int J Vitamin Res 39: 447–456.

9. Nakamura R, Littarru GP, Folkers K (1972): Abstract for the 9th Annual National Meeting of the Reticuloendothelial Society, Austin, Texas, December 5–8, 1972.

10. Bliznakov EG, Casey AC, Premuzic E (1970): Experientia 26: 953–954.

11. Casey AC, Bliznakov EG (1972): Chem-Biol Interactions 5: 1–12.

12. Bliznakov EG (1973): Proc Natl Acad Sci USA 70: 390–394.

13. Bliznakov EG, Casey AC, Kishi T, Kishi H, Folkers K (1975): Int J Vitamin Nutr Res 45: 388–395.

14. Bliznakov EG (1977): In Folkers K, Yamamura, Y (eds): "Biomedical and Clinical Aspects of Coenzyme Q." New York: Elsevier/North-Holland Biomedical Press, Vol I, pp 73–83.

15. Bliznakov EG, Watnabe T, Saji S, Folkers K (1978): J Med 9: 337–346.

16. Folkers K, Shizukuishi S, Takemura K, Drzewoski J, Richardson P, Ellis J, Kuzell WC (1982): Res Commun Chem Path Pharm 38: 335–338.

17. Ye C, Folkers K, Tamagawa H, Pfeifer C (1988): BioFactors, submitted.

18. Komorowski J, Muratsu K, Nara Y, Willis R, Folkers K (1988): BioFactors 1: 67–69.

Vitamins and Cancer Prevention, pages 111–127
Published 1991 Wiley-Liss, Inc.

| 9 | # The Future of Nutrition Research in Cancer Prevention |

Peter Greenwald, M.D., Dr.P.H.

INTRODUCTION

With the exception of smoking, dietary habits are the single most significant lifestyle factor in cancer risk [1,2]. This means that there should be a major potential for reducing cancer incidence in the general population through dietary modification. The development and implementation of nutrition-based cancer intervention strategies targeted at the general population

Division of Cancer Prevention and Control, National Cancer Institute, National Institutes of Health, Bethesda, Maryland 20892

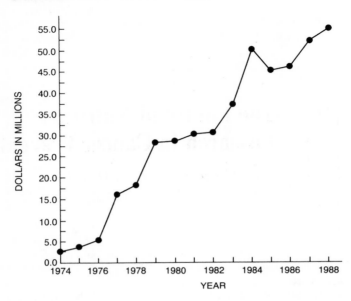

Fig. 1.   National Cancer Institute nutrition research budget.

or specific high risk groups can have a beneficial impact on public health. Despite the incomplete knowledge of fundamental nutritional mechanisms that affect cancer, there are presently enough research leads to justify an optimistic and aggressive approach to nutrition research related to cancer. For this reason, the National Cancer Institute (NCI) has greatly increased its commitment to diet, nutrition, and cancer research. Over the past 15 years, the nutrition research budget at NCI has grown from an annual expenditure of $2.5 million in 1974 to more than $55.0 million in 1988 (Fig. 1). Sufficient evidence, outlined below, has already accumulated to develop and test several hypotheses in clinical cancer prevention (intervention) trials with selected macronutrients and micronutrients. Other research efforts are directed at developing chemopreventive (cancer-inhibiting) compounds from natural and synthetic sources and promoting a host of nutrition research activities.

THE ROLE OF SPECIFIC DIETARY FACTORS ON CANCER RISK

A large body of epidemiological evidence provides consistent support for a relationship between specific dietary components and the development of certain cancers, notably those of endocrine or digestive system origin (breast, prostate, colon, and stomach). Vitamins A, C, E, carotenoids, selenium, calcium, fiber, and a number of nonnutritive components are hypothesized to contribute alone, or in combination, to the apparent cancer-preventive effect of certain food groups identified in dietary recall studies. Both epidemiological and laboratory research identify high intakes of dietary fat as cancer promoting. Some of the evidence for the role of specific dietary constituents on cancer development is discussed below. The reader is referred to several recent reviews for a more comprehensive presentation [2–6].

Fat

Fat has been studied more extensively and is associated more frequently with various cancers than any other dietary factor. Human population data show strong positive correlations between total dietary fat and caloric intake and cancer incidence, particularly for the endocrine-related cancers of the breast and prostate, and also colorectal cancer [3].

Comparisons of dietary fat intake by country indicate, for example, that populations with the highest per capita fat consumption have the highest breast cancer mortality: Denmark has a fivefold greater rate of mortality from breast cancer than Japan [7]. Migration data among women from areas with low breast cancer rates to areas with higher rates show increased breast cancer risk with migration. This trend is seen among Japanese women migrating to Hawaii [8] and Italian women migrating to Australia [9]. Time trend data, in which increasing fat intake among certain population groups over time is measured, also reveal a correlation between dietary fat and breast cancer incidence [10]. Prentice [11] recently showed that the strong international correlation with breast cancer rates holds for total calories from fat, but not for nonfat calories.

Dietary fat is consistently observed to be a tumor promotor in experimental studies. Restricted caloric intake was found by Tannenbaum and Silverstone [12] to inhibit tumor development in a series of studies using mouse mammary tumor models; increasing levels of dietary fat increased tumor yield and size. Animals fed high-fat diets ad libitum exhibited tumors earlier and with greater frequency than animals fed low-fat diets. Many other animal studies have since confirmed that dietary fat increases mammary tumor incidence or multiplicity or decreases tumor latency [13].

The type of dietary fat implicated in cancer promotion is a current research focus. Both the degree of saturation and chain length can affect the impact of dietary fat on tumorigenesis; olive oil and medium chain triglycerides derived from coconut oil are reported to lack promoting ability in mammary tumor models [14]. Studies in humans suggest that high saturated fat (SFA) intake is associated with increased incidence for some cancers. In animals, omega-6 polyunsaturated fatty acids (PUFA) and high SFA intake increase cancer risk [15,16]. The converse is found with fish oils containing eicosopentaenoic acid (an omega-3 PUFA) or oleic acid, a monounsaturated fatty acid (MUFA) from olive oil, which tend to inhibit carcinogenesis in animals. This may explain the low incidence of breast and colon cancer in Eskimos whose main fat source is fish and in some Mediterranean peoples whose main fat source is olive oil [17]. Available data, however, do not yet permit a clear distinction to be made between the effect of different types of fat on cancer risk.

Thus data from both experimental and human correlational studies strongly support the association between dietary fat and breast cancer. Although some well-designed case-control and cohort studies do conclude that there is no association [18–20], these divergent results may be due to the limitations and inadequacies inherent in the conduct of nutritionally related epidemiological research. Dietary assessment techniques are inexact and subject to a wide range of error, and many cohorts surveyed have only a very small variation in their dietary fat intake level. As emphasized in a recent overview [4], intensive efforts to design better studies are needed to objectively test the biologically plausible dietary fat–breast cancer hypothesis.

Fiber

The hypothesis that dietary fiber may be protective against colorectal cancer originally stems from the observation that in Africa, where the intake of dietary fiber is very high, there is a relative lack of cancer of the large intestine and other chronic gastrointestinal diseases common in Western countries [21]. As a result, numerous studies have explored a possible protective role by fiber. A recent review of 40 epidemiologic studies indicated an inverse association between total dietary fiber intake and colon cancer incidence in 32 of the 40 studies [22].

Comparisons between populations with differing colon cancer incidence rates but similar levels of fat intake have been made [2] among people from north and south India [23], Denmark and Finland [24], and rural Finland and New York [25]. In these studies the lower risk populations had higher fiber intakes. A study in New Zealand, however, showed that Maoris have lower colon cancer rates, despite lower fiber and higher fat intake, than whites [26]. Although results from numerous case-control, international, and within-country correlational studies generally reflect an inverse or protective association between dietary fiber and colon cancer risk, several studies show no association or a direct association [27]. Differences may exist because dietary fibers from different food sources are heterogeneous mixtures of components, such as cellulose, hemicelluloses, pectins, gums, and lignin, and therefore may have varying physiological effects. In addition, fiber components are difficult to accurately quantitate in foods. It has also been difficult to separate the effects of fiber from other dietary constituents (e.g., total calories, fats, vitamins, minerals, and nonnutritive components of fruits and vegetables) and nondietary factors (e.g., socioeconomic status). A genetic susceptibility, inherited or acquired, to colon cancer in certain populations is also possible and only recently amenable to detection [28,29]. In a recent analysis of colorectal tumor specimens the accumulation of genetic alterations paralleled clinical tumor development [29].

In laboratory studies, the effect of various components of fiber on chemically induced colon cancer in rodents is also inconsistent [30]. Cancer inhibitory or enhancing effects are variously reported by different authors for the same fiber source. Results in these experiments can be influenced markedly by experimental variables such as the type of fiber, the chemical carcinogen, other dietary factors (especially fat), and the route and dose of fiber–carcinogen administration. Of the many fiber sources tested, wheat bran, cellulose, and citrus fiber are generally found to inhibit colon cancer tumor yield or size [27].

Mechanisms proposed for the inhibitory role of fiber in colorectal carcinogenesis include reducing fecal mutagen concentrations by increasing fecal bulk, reducing the length of exposure by colonic mucosa to fecal mutagens by enhanced fecal transit time, and inhibiting fecal mutagen synthesis through fiber-induced changes in colonic pH or bacterial metabolism.

Micronutrients

Numerous epidemiologic studies have shown that daily consumption of vegetables and fruits is associated with decreased risk of lung, bladder, esophagus, and stomach cancers [3]. A variety of components in these foods may be responsible alone or together for the decreased cancer risk in these studies. For example, Ziegler [31] reviewed the epidemiologic evidence that carotenoids reduce cancer risk. In both prospective and retrospective studies, low intakes of fruits and vegetables containing carotenoids or vitamin A are associated with an increased risk of lung and certain other cancers. Low levels of beta-carotene intake in smokers are strongly correlated with subsequent development of lung cancer [32], and several studies report that serum levels of vitamin A or carotenoids are related to subsequent cancer risk [33–35].

Several studies have explored the potential chemopreventive effects of carotenoids on experimentally induced tumors; however, there is little evidence that these compounds have an inherent activity independent of their ultimate conversion to vitamin A [36]. In contrast, studies with vitamin A and other related retinoids consistently demonstrate that these compounds can interfere with the progression of cancer [37]. Among the inhibitory effects found for retinoids are regression of chemically induced tumors [38]; arrest or suppression of malignant transformation [39–41]; and induction of terminal differentiation from a malignant to a nonmalignant phenotype [42,43]. The synthesis of retinoid derivatives to minimize toxicity and enhance chemopreventive activity is generating more compounds for testing and evaluation. One such compound, isotretinoin, was demonstrated in a prospective intervention trial to be effective in preventing or delaying new skin cancer development in patients with xeroderma pigmentosum [44].

Several epidemiological studies suggest an inverse relationship between vitamin C containing foods and cancer of the stomach and esophagus [40,41]. Although findings are inconsistent for cancers of the colon, rectum, and lung, frequent consumption of primary sources of vitamin C (fruits and vegetables) is strongly associated with a protective effect against lung cancer [45,46]. The potentially protective effects of other factors in vitamin C rich foods (beta-carotene and vitamin A) make conclusions about this vitamin and cancer difficult. However, ascorbic acid does inhibit nitrosamine formation from secondary and higher amines in combination with nitrites in humans [47,48]. In animal models, vitamin C inhibits the development of some cancers, such as dermal neoplasms [49], renal carcinoma [50], and colorectal tumors [51].

In addition to reducing the formation of carcinogenic nitrosamines in the gut, it is postulated that ascorbic acid may inhibit carcinogenesis by reducing other highly reactive endogenous compounds such as superoxide radicals. Thus, like beta-carotene, vitamin C may act as an antioxidant. Vitamin E, another important tissue antioxidant, is another proposed preventive compound; however, this vitamin is also difficult to study epidemiologically because it is widespread in foods, and concentrations can vary widely within individual foodstuffs. In one study [43] serum vitamin E (and beta-carotene) levels were lower in persons who later developed squamous-cell carcinoma of the lung compared with controls, a finding that differs from a similar study on cancer risk by Willett et al. [33].

Other micronutrients for which there is epidemiological or laboratory evidence for cancer inhibition include riboflavin, selenium, zinc, and calcium [39,52–61]. It should be remembered that nutrient deprivation enhances susceptibility to disease and that conclusions from studies, both animal and human, that examine the role of micronutrients under conditions of deprivation may not be directly applicable to situations in which the organism is not stressed in this manner.

NCI NUTRITION RESEARCH PROGRAMS

The expanding nutrition research programs at NCI are designed to emphasize the objective testing of hypotheses developed from epidemiological and laboratory leads related to diet and cancer and to promote the accumulation of more detailed knowledge on nutrient activities and interactions and foodstuff composition. This research is undertaken primarily by the Cancer Prevention Research Program, which comprises a diet and cancer research program, a chemoprevention research program, and nutrition-related health promotion activities.

Diet and Cancer Research

The major thrust of the diet and cancer research program is to identify, test, and implement cancer reduction strategies based on dietary modification. This overall objective is being achieved through extramural basic and clinical studies and by applied nutrition research and nutrition coordination activities within NCI and other organizations. Current research includes developing methodology to analyze dietary fiber, vitamin A, and carotenoids in foods; studying the metabolism and physicochemical effects of fiber, retinoids, and carotenoids in humans; planning and coordinating the women's clinical feasibility trial on the role of dietary fat in breast cancer; and sponsoring workshops to review the state of the science in such areas as fiber and colon cancer and diet and gastric cancer.

Several ongoing projects are concerned with establishing a data base on food component quantity, nutritional composition, absorption, and metabolism. This work includes a cooperative project with the Food and Drug Administration and several European countries to establish an international food component data base that will provide information on the content of nutrients, additives, contaminants, and naturally occurring substances in food. Recently, NCI has approved the establishment of an Intramural Cancer Nutrition Research Laboratory and created a new Laboratory of Nutritional and Molecular Regulation. These facilities will greatly enhance the ability of the Cancer Prevention Research Program to conduct multidisciplinary research in the nutritional sciences, including human feeding studies and nutritional epidemiology.

The design and conduct of clinical trials to study the relationship between dietary factors and cancer is another important area of research. Studies are being planned to clarify the relationship between dietary fat, total calories, and net energy balance with the development of breast cancer and to elucidate the relationship between blood and tissue level micronutrients. To test the fat–breast cancer hypothesis, a clinical intervention trial designed to detect a decreased incidence of breast cancer in high-risk women maintained on a low-fat diet (20% of calories) was designed by a multidisciplinary group of scientists, requiring more than 30,000 subjects to be followed for up to 10 years. The feasibility of the trial, including methodology for subject recruitment, nutritional counseling, and compliance monitoring, was demonstrated in a pilot study. Although implementation of the full-scale trial was abandoned due to controversy over aspects of the study design and the large commitment of resources, the pilot study population continues to be monitored.

Chemoprevention Research

In addition to dietary modification schemes, NCI is working to identify compounds with activity as cancer preventives and to develop them as supplements for use in clinical prevention strategies. Micronutrients (as opposed to whole foods or macronutrients), naturally occurring chemicals in food or other natural products, and synthetics are under evaluation. More than 600 chemopreventive compounds are under consideration for development, with about 50 agents or agent combinations currently under study in a preclinical setting. These candidate chemopreventives are derived from a wide range of sources, represent varied chemical structures, and exhibit diverse physiological effects: the micronutrients vitamins A, C, and E, selenium, molybdenum, calcium; the natural products carotenoids, terpenoids, isothiocyanates, flavonoids, and phenolics; and the synthetics Oltipraz, piroxicam, tamoxifen, difluoromethyl ornithine, and several retinoid derivatives. Proposed mechanisms of action for chemopreventives are as diverse as the structures represented in the above list. Inhibition of neoplastic initiation or progression is postulated to proceed from such actions as inhibition of the metabolic activation of chemical carcinogens, inactivation of reactive genotoxic species, and inhibition of signal transduction pathways crucial for neoplastic progression (antiinflammatory agents, prostaglandin synthetase inhibitors, hormone analogs, etc.).

Conducted in a series of stages, the chemoprevention program screens potentially useful compounds in a preclinical setting followed by the selection of promising candidate inhibitors for testing in human intervention studies.

Clinical Intervention Trials

The NCI is currently supporting 19 clinical intervention trials designed to test the ability of selected micronutrients, fiber, or certain synthetics to reduce the incidence of cancer in the population at large or in individuals at high risk for developing cancer at a given site. Each of these is a controlled, prospective, randomized trial—the most desirable experimental technique for testing a human preventive intervention strategy.

Beta-carotene supplements are being evaluated in a healthy population (U. S. physician's study) and in high-risk subjects. A collaborative U. S.–Finland study is investigating the effectiveness of beta-carotene and vitamin E as a lung cancer preventive in smokers. A series of vitamin and mineral supplement combinations is being tested in a Chinese population at high risk for developing esophageal cancer. The role of fiber and calcium in preventing colon cancer or precancerous colorectal polyps is under study in several separate clinical paradigms.

Since 1980, there has been a substantial increase in the number of pre-clinical and clinical studies with nutritionally derived cancer preventives. In 1990, NCI will consider approximately 200 new prospective chemopreventive agents for screening, many of which are natural products from food sources. Clinical research in both chemoprevention and dietary modification is expected in the future to emphasize trials that utilize an intermediate endpoint of cancer risk (rather than cancer incidence) for evaluating the effectiveness of newly proposed intervention strategies. The development and use of intermediate endpoint markers, such as cervical dysplasia, to predict future cancer incidence will enable investigators to design clinical trials with much smaller populations and shorter follow-up times [62].

DIETARY GUIDELINES

While the importance of diet in reducing cancer risk is being further established by current research, it is prudent, based on existing findings, to propose interim guidelines to increase intake of fruits, vegetables, and whole grains (high-fiber foods) while decreasing the intake of fat and maintaining desirable weight. Two recent reports, Diet and Health [2] prepared by the Food and Nutrition Board of the National Academy of Sciences (NAS), and the *Surgeon General's Report on Nutrition and Health* [63] make similar dietary recommendations for decreasing chronic disease risk based upon critical reviews of the available data. Both reports emphasize diets rich in prospective chemopreventive factors and recommend reducing factors that may be cancer promoting.

The highest priority is given to reducing fat intake. Americans currently consume about 36–38% of their total daily calories from fat [64,65]. The recommendation that Americans reduce that percentage to 30% or less to reduce risk for cancer and other diseases has been made by many expert groups, including NCI [66], the American Cancer Society [67], the American Heart Association [68], and the USDA [69], as well as NAS [2,70], based upon the strong scientific evidence concerning dietary fats and human health. The Surgeon General's Report, although strongly recommending a reduction in fat consumption, does not specify the amount of decrease.

In view of the evidence that dietary fiber may moderate the effects of fat and considering the consistency of the epidemiological data that inversely associate dietary fiber intake with colon cancer, some groups, including NCI, recommend that the U. S. adult population increase dietary fiber intake from a variety of food sources. The recent report by the NAS states that at present the evidence for the association between cancer risk and fiber intake is unclear and makes its recommendations not specifically addressing fiber [2].

Although these and other guidelines (such as limiting alcohol consumption) reflect current knowledge and are based upon the best available scientific data, determination of the precise contribution of diet to overall cancer risk is not yet possible. Understanding the exact manner in which diet affects tumor incidence and promotion and devising strategies for altering this process are the continuing challenges of nutrition-based cancer prevention research. Meanwhile, the most sensible and beneficial course of action is to promote adherence to the interim dietary guidelines until more definitive recommendations can be made. The evidence is sufficiently convincing that the guidelines have a high likelihood of health benefit with no discernible risk while being consistent with good nutritional practices.

FUTURE DIRECTIONS FOR DIET AND CANCER PREVENTION RESEARCH

The NAS Diet and Health Committee, having conducted a critical and comprehensive survey of the role of nutritional factors in disease, has identified a series of research needs that apply directly to diet and cancer research. These topic areas are of current and continuing interest to NCI and will in the future be the subject of increasing emphasis.

There are many fundamental questions that remain to be answered before the role of nutritional factors in the development of cancer is clearly understood. An important research need is identifying foods and dietary components that alter cancer risk and elucidating their mechanisms of action. The full contribution of any nutrient, alone or in combination, with respect to cancer risk has not been completely ascertained. Although certain compounds are often labeled as "antioxidants" or "free radical scavengers," this is usually a reflection of chemical activity in vitro, and can only suggest, but not establish, that such activity occurs in vivo to affect cancer initiation or promotion. Furthermore, the interaction of dietary influences on other lifestyle and genetic factors that contribute to the occurrence of cancer has not been well delineated. The biological activity of nonnutritive compounds is even less well understood than those that we have long known are required for health. Many compounds routinely consumed in food sources are mutagenic, carcinogenic, or cancer preventive in laboratory assays [5,71]. The contribution of these factors to a dietary influence on cancer also requires scrutiny.

With regard to specific dietary constituents, the role of different types of dietary fat (SFA, PUFA, MUFA) on cancer risk is unclear, as are possible mechanisms through which dietary fat can influence the process of carcinogenesis. The numerous combinations of chemicals that we term "dietary fiber" have not been fully agreed upon, and the biological effects of specific fiber components need further clarification. The manner in which natural fiber or fiber supplements may alter the metabolism or absorption of other nutrients is only now being investigated. The NCI has supported research on the analysis of dietary fiber and fiber components of food. Methods are under development that will improve the accuracy and reliability of analytical procedures for fiber and fiber components.

Identifying the adverse and beneficial effects of dietary components remains to be accomplished. It is necessary to determine in a more rigorous manner the optimal ranges of intake for a given nutrient to allow for more definitive and precise dietary recommendations. It is possible that selected high-risk individuals might benefit from dietary interventions at levels of intake well above the Recommended Daily Allowance, although this is not established at present. Improved dietary assessment techniques must be developed. Better methods for data collection, quantifying dietary exposures and effects, and data analysis are needed to more accurately and precisely conduct population surveys and clinical trials. For example, the quality and comprehensiveness of the food composition data bases used in survey research need improvement, specifically those used to estimate the vitamin A and fiber content of foods. Innovative methods for dietary assessment in population samples, such as identifying meaningful and practical biological markers of exposure, may yield more reliable estimates of intake and less inconsistency among studies.

Besides identifying markers of dietary exposure, there is a pressing need to identify early indicators that can predict the emergence of cancer, and gene markers that can identify high-risk subgroups in the population. Greater application of these techniques in the design and conduct of nutritional studies will narrow the range of variables under study and yield research designs with more definitive outcomes.

Carefully designed intervention studies are needed to demonstrate with more certainty that diet is a significant and controllable factor in cancer etiology. Such trials should be planned on the basis of epidemiologic and experimental evidence, identifying the best study population and dietary modification most warranting investigation. For example, the feasibility of intervention studies to determine the effects of reduced fat intake on the incidence of common cancers, especially breast and colorectal and possibly prostate cancer, in a defined population needs consideration. Large sample sizes and long-term follow-up are required for such studies.

Social and behavioral research is needed to better motivate change in dietary habits. This knowledge is necessary to design effective public health programs aimed at reducing cancer risk. Furthermore, improved technologies, such as those developing in the fields of agriculture and food science, are needed to increase the availability of foods that conform to established dietary guidelines and allow people to follow beneficial dietary practices.

HEALTH IMPLICATIONS OF THE CHANGING FOOD SUPPLY

Future research directions discussed above focus on improving our knowledge of the interrelationships between diet and cancer. There is also a need for an awareness and understanding of present changes in the food supply and the implications of these changes on diet and health. Past technologies, such as canning and refrigeration, which reduced food contaminants and ensured a year-round safe and more varied food supply, are believed to have contributed to the decline in mortality and incidence rates for gastric cancer worldwide over the past 50 years [72]. Recent developments in agriculture and food science, including agricultural and food biotechnology, are having a dramatic effect on the proliferation of available marketplace foods. For example, the number of shelf items in the average supermarket for the years 1928, 1983, and 1988 increased from 867 to 16,000 to 24,000 items, respectively [73]. The extensive number of new foods introduced by these new technologies may have profound health implications.

A favorable development in the food industry driven by consumer demand is an emphasis on lower fat foods. Many low-fat counterparts for commonly consumed high-fat foods are now available. Recently developed fat substitutes, such as Olestra® and Simplesse®, may reduce the percentage of fat in numerous oil-based and dairy products [74,75]. Sharp reductions have been made in the total fat content of market livestock through breeding, genetic improvement, and the use of growth hormones [76,77]. Also, there is a greater availability of poultry and fish products.

Another favorable trend is the increased availability and variety of fiber-rich foods (e.g., fruits, vegetables, and grains) offered in the marketplace. In addition to their beneficial nutritive and nonnutritive constituents, these foods have value in displacing high-fat foods in the diet. Ready-to-eat breakfast cereals, pasta, and whole-wheat bread consumption have shown striking increases since the mid-1960s [78]. Also, advances in food biotechnology are providing us with greater yields of high-quality fruits and vegetables, with improved disease resistance and nutritional content [79]. For example, new germination techniques can produce a 10-fold increase in the vitamin C content of peas and beans [80]. *P. fluorescens,* modified to produce a toxin, can be used as a microbial insecticide for corn [76]. Also, the knowledge gained by investigators studying the regulation of ripening enzymes will lead to the availability of tomatoes that taste vine-ripened, yet do not soften before reaching the market [81].

CONCLUSIONS

It is evident that dietary modifications can have a major impact on public health and cancer incidence in particular. The NCI attaches great importance to supporting research to further identify chemopreventive factors in foods and more rigorously establish the links between diet and cancer. Such knowledge can provide a framework for industry, government, and an informed public to work together in creating and utilizing a food supply that promotes optimal health. The need for such knowledge becomes even more pressing, as the time may come when clinicians can predict individual patient risk for developing cancer and need to be able to offer more than tentative prevention strategies.

REFERENCES

1. Doll R, Peto R (1981): The causes of cancer: quantitative estimates of avoidable risks of cancer in the United States today. J Natl Cancer Inst 66:1192–1308.
2. National Academy of Sciences. National Research Council. Food and Nutrition Board. Diet and health: implications for reducing chronic disease risk. Council on Life Sciences, 1989. National Academy Press, Washington, DC.
3. National Academy of Sciences. National Research Council. Committee on Diet, Nutrition and Cancer. Diet, nutrition, and cancer. Assembly of Life Sciences, 1982. National Academy Press, Washington, DC.
4. Schatzkin A, Greenwald P, Byar DP, Clifford CK (1989): The dietary fat-breast cancer hypothesis is alive. J Am Med Assoc 261(22):3284–3287.
5. Bertram JS, Kolonel LN, Meyskens FL (1987): Rationale and strategies for chemoprevention of cancer in humans. Cancer Res 47(6):3012–3031.
6. Vogel VG, McPherson RS (1989): Dietary epidemiology of colon cancer: new perspectives in large bowel cancer. Hematology/Oncology Clinics of North America 3:35–63.
7. Wynder EL, MacCormick F, Hill P, Cohen LA, Chan PC, Weisburger JH (1976): Nutrition and the etiology and prevention of breast cancer. Cancer Detect Prev 1:293–310.
8. Dunn JE (1977): Breast cancer among American Japanese in the San Francisco Bay area. NCI Monogr 47:157–160.
9. McMichael AJ, Giles GG (1988): Cancer in migrants to Australia: extending the descriptive epidemiologic data. Cancer Res 48:751–756.
10. Kurihara M, Aoki K, Tominaga S (1984): Cancer mortality statistics in the world. Nagoya, Japan: University of Nagoya Press.
11. Prentice RL, Kakar F, Hursting S, Sheppard L, Klein R, Kushi LH (1988): Aspects of the rationale for the Women's Health Trial. J Natl Cancer Inst 80:802–814.
12. Tannenbaum A, Silverstone H (1953): Nutrition in relation to cancer. Adv Cancer Res 1:451–501.

13. Carroll K (1980): Lipids and carcinogenesis. J Environ Path Tox 3:250–271.
14. Cohen LA (1987): Dietary fat and mammary cancer. In Reddy BS, Cohen LA (eds): "Diet, nutrition, and cancer: a critical evaluation." Boca Raton, FL: CRC Press, pp 76–100.
15. Ip C, Carter CA, Ip MM (1985): Requirement of essential fatty acid for mammary tumorigenesis in the rat. Cancer Res 45:1997–2001.
16. Ip C (1987): Fat and essential fatty acid in mamnary carcinogenesis. Am J Clin Nutr 45:218–224.
17. Kinsella JE (1986): Food components with potential therapeutic benefits: the n-3 polyunsaturated fatty acids of fish oils. Food Tech 40:89–97.
18. Goodwin PJ, Boyd NF (1987): Critical appraisal of the evidence that dietary fat intake is related to breast cancer risk in humans. J Natl Cancer Inst 79:473–485.
19. Willett WC, Stampfer MJ, Colditz GA, Rosner BA, Hennekens CH, Speizer FE (1987): Dietary fat and the risk of breast cancer. N Engl J Med 316:22–28.
20. Jones DY, Schatzkin A, Green SB, Block G, Brinton LA, Ziegler RG, Hoover R, Taylor PR (1987): Dietary fat and breast cancer in the National Health and Nutrition Examination Survey. I. Epidemiologic follow-up study. J Natl Cancer Inst 79:465–471.
21. Burkitt DP (1971): Epidemiology of cancer of the colon and rectum. Cancer 28:3–13.
22. Greenwald P, Lanza E, Eddy GA (1987): Dietary fiber in the reduction of colon cancer risk. J Am Diet Assoc 87(9):1178–1188.
23. Malhotra SL (1977): Dietary factors in a study of cancer colon from cancer registry, with special reference to the role of saliva, milk, and fermented milk products and vegetable fibre. Med Hypotheses 3:122–126.
24. Jensen OM, MacLennan R, Wahrendorf J (1982): Diet, bowel function, fecal characteristics, and large bowel cancer in Denmark and Finland. Nutr Cancer 4:5–19.
25. Reddy BS, Hedges AR, Laakso K, Wynder EL (1978): Metabolic epidemiology of large bowel cancer: fecal bulk and constituents of high-risk North American and low-risk Finnish population. Cancer 42:2832–2838.
26. Smith AH, Pearce NE, Joseph JG (1985): Major colorectal aetiological hypotheses do not explain mortality trends among Maori and non-Maori New Zealanders. Int J Epidemiol 14:79–85.
27. Pilch SM (ed) (1987): Physiological effects and health consequences of dietary fiber. Life Sciences Research Office, FASEB, Bethesda, MD, pp 118–135.
28. Bodmer WF, Bailey CJ, Bodmer J, Bussey HJR, Ellis A, Gorman P, Lucibello FC, Murday VA, Rider SH, Scambler P, Sheer P, Solomon E, Spurr WK (1987): Localization of the gene for familial adenomatous polyposis on chromosome 5. Nature 328:614–616.
29. Vogelstein B, Fearon ER, Hamilton SR, Kern SE, Preisinger AC, Leppert M, Nakamura Y, White R, Smits AMM, Bos JL (1988): Genetic alterations during colorectal-tumor development. N Engl J Med 319:525–532.
30. Reddy BS (1987): Diet and colon cancer: evidence from human and animal model studies. In Reddy BS, Cohen LA (eds): "Diet, nutrition, and cancer: a critical evaluation." Boca Raton, FL: CRC Press, pp 47–65.
31. Ziegler RG (1989): A review of epidemiologic evidence that carotenoids reduce the risk of cancer. J Nutr 119(1):116–122.
32. Shekelle RB, Lepper M, Liu S, Maliza C, Raynor WJ Jr, Rossof AH, Paul O, Shryock AM, Stamler J (1981): Dietary vitamin A and risk of cancer in the Western Electric study. Lancet 2:1186–1190.
33. Willett W, Polk R, Underwood BA, Stampfer MJ, Pressel S, Rasner B, Taylor JO, Schneider K, Hames CG (1984): Relation of serum vitamin A and E and carotenoids to the risk of cancer. N Engl J Med 310:430–434.

34. Kark JD, Smith AH, Switzer BR, Hames CC (1981): Serum vitamin A (retinol) and cancer incidence in Evans County, Georgia. J Natl Cancer Inst 66:7–16.
35. Wald N, Idle M, Boreham J, Bailey A (1980): Low serum-vitamin A and subsequent risk of cancer: preliminary results of a prospective study. Lancet 2:813–815.
36. Peto R (1983): The marked difference between carotenoids and retinoids: methodological implications for biochemical epidemiology. Cancer Surv 2:327–340.
37. Sporn MB, Roberts AB (1983): Role of retinoids in differentiation and carcinogenesis. Cancer Res 43:3034–3040.
38. Carr BI (1985): Chemical carcinogens and inhibitors of carcinogenesis in the human diet. Cancer 55:218–224.
39. Schrauzer GN, White DA, Schneider CJ (1977): Cancer mortality correlation studies. III. Statistical associations with dietary selenium intakes. Bioinorgan Chem 7:23–31.
40. Mettlin C, Graham S, Priore R, Marshall J, Swanson M (1981): Diet and cancer of the esophagus. Nutr Cancer 2:143–147.
41. Haenszel N, Correa P (1975): Development in the epidemiology of stomach cancer over the past decade. Cancer Res 35:3452–3459.
42. Mirvish SS, Wallcave L, Eagen M, Shubik P (1972): Ascorbate-nitrite reaction: possible means of blocking the formation of carcinogenic N-nitroso compounds. Science 177: 65–68.
43. Menkes MS, Comstock GW, Vuilleumier JP, Helsing KJ, Rider AA, Brooksmeyer R (1986): Serum beta-carotene, vitamins A and E, selenium and the risk of lung cancer. N Engl J Med 315:1250–1254.
44. Kraemer KH, DiGiovanna JJ, Moshell AN, Tarone RE, Peck GL (1988): Prevention of skin cancer in xeroderma pigmentosum. N Engl J Med 1988;318:1633–1637.
45. Hirayama T (1979): Diet and cancer. Nutr Cancer 1:67–81.
46. MacLennan R, DaCosta J, Day NE, Law CH, Ng YK, Shanmugaratum K (1977): Risk factors for lung cancer in Singapore Chinese, a population with high female incidence rates. Int J Cancer 20:854–860.
47. Mirvish SS (1975): Blocking the formation of N-nitroso compounds with ascorbic acid in vitro and in vivo. Ann NY Acad Sci 258:175–180.
48. Raineri R, Weisburger JH (1975): Reduction of gastric carcinogens with ascorbic acid. Ann NY Acad Sci 258:181–189.
49. Dunhan WB, Zuckerkandl E, Reynolds R, Willoughby R, Marcuson R, Barth R, Pauling L (1982): Effects of intake of L-ascorbic acid on the incidence of dermal neoplasms induced by ultraviolet light. Proc Natl Acad Sci USA 79:7532–7536.
50. Liehr JG, Wheeler WJ (1983): Inhibition of estrogen-induced renal carcinoma in Syrian hamsters by vitamin C. Cancer Res 43:4638–4642.
51. Basu TK, Schorah CJ (1982): Vitamin C in health and disease. Westport, CT: AVI.
52. Thurnham DI, Zheng SF, Munoz N, Crespi M, Grassi A, Hambridge KM, Chai TF (1985): Comparison of riboflavin, vitamin A, and zinc status of Chinese populations at high and low risk for esophageal cancer. Nutr Cancer 7:131–143.
53. Foy H, Kondi A (1984): The vulnerable esophagus: riboflavin deficiency and squamous cell dysplasia of the skin and the esophagus. J Natl Cancer Inst 72:941–948.
54. van Rensburg SJ, Hall JM, Gathercole PS (1986): Inhibition of esophageal carcinogenesis in corn-fed rats by riboflavin, nicotinic acid, selenium, molybdenum, zinc, and magnesium. Nutr Cancer 8:163–170.
55. Shamberger RJ, Tylko SA, Willis CE (1976): Antioxidants and cancer. VI. Selenium and age-adjusted human cancer mortality. Arch Environ Health 31:231–235.
56. Beach RS, Gershwin ME, Hurley LS (1981): Dietary zinc modulation of Moloney sarcoma virus oncogenesis. Cancer Res 41:552–559.

57. Fernandes G, Nair M, Onoe K, Tanaka T, Floyd R, Good RA (1979): Impairment of cell-mediated immunity functions by dietary zinc deficiency in mice. Proc Natl Acad Sci USA 76:457–461.
58. Golden MHN, Golden BE, Harland PSEG, Jackson AA (1978): Zinc and immunocompetence in protein-energy malnutrition. Lancet 1:1226–1228.
59. Hurley LS (1981): Teratogenic aspects of manganese, zinc, and copper nutrition. Physiol Rev 61:249–295.
60. Garland C, Shekelle RB, Barrett-Conner E, Criqui MH, Rossof AH, Paul O (1985): Dietary vitamin D and calcium and risk of colorectal cancer. A 19-year prospective study in men. Lancet 1:307–309.
61. Slattery ML, Sorenson AW, Ford MH (1988): Dietary calcium intake as a mitigating factor in colon cancer. Am J Epidemiol 128:504–514.
62. Greenwald P (1989): Principles of carcinogenesis: dietary factors. In DeVita VT, Jr, Hillman S, Rosenberg SA (eds): "Cancer, principles and practice of oncology," 3rd ed. Philadelphia: Lippincott, pp 167–180.
63. US Department of Health and Human Services, Public Health Service (1988): The Surgeon General's report on nutrition and health. DHHS (PHS) publication No. 88-50211. Washington, DC: Government Printing Office.
64. USDA (1986): Nationwide food consumption continuous survey of food intake by individuals: men 19–50 years, 1 day, 1985. Report No. 85-3, pp 1–46.
65. USDA (1987): Nationwide food consumption continuous survey of food intake by individuals: women 19–50 years and their children 1–5 years, 1 day, 1986. Report No. 86-1, pp 1–46.
66. Butrum RR, Clifford CK, Lanza E (1988): NCI dietary guidelines: rationale. Am J Clin Nutr 48:888–895.
67. American Cancer Society (1985): Nutrition, common sense, and cancer. New York: American Cancer Society (No. 2096-LE).
68. American Heart Association (1985): The American Heart Association diet—an eating plan for healthy Americans. Dallas, TX: American Heart Association, (No. 51-018-B[SA]).
69. USDA (1985): Nutrition and your health: dietary guidelines for Americans, 2nd ed. Washington, DC: U.S. Government Printing Office, (Home and garden bulletin No. 232).
70. Palmer S, Bakshi K (1983): Diet, nutrition and cancer: interim dietary guidelines. J Natl Cancer Inst 70(6):1153–1170.
71. Ames BN (1983): Dietary carcinogens and anticarcinogens. Science 221:1256–1264.
72. Howson CP, Hiyama T, Wynder EL (1986): The decline in gastric cancer: epidemiology of an unplanned triumph. Epidemiol Rev 8:1–27.
73. Borra S (1988): Considerations for implementing dietary guidelines in the retail food industry. Presentation to the National Academy of Sciences, Food and Nutrition Board. Guidelines on diets and health: implications and strategies for implementation.
74. Toma RB, Curtis DJ, Sobotor C (1988): Sucrose polyester: its metabolic role and possible future applications. Food Tech 42(1):93–95.
75. Anonymous (1988): Fat substitute for dairy and oil-based products. Food Tech 42(4):96–97.
76. Food and Drug Administration (1988): Office of Planning and Evaluation and the Center for Food Safety and Applied Nutrition. Food biotechnology: present and future. Vols I and II. Washington, DC.
77. Breidenstein BC (1988): Changes in consumer attitudes toward red meat and their effect on marketing strategy. Food Tech 42(1):112–114.
78. Leveille GA (1988): Current attitude and behavior trends regarding consumption of grains. Food Tech 42(1):110–111.

79. Teutonico RA, Knorr D (1985): Impact of biotechnology on nutritional quality of food plants. Food Tech 39(10):127–134.
80. Fordham JR, Wells CE, Chen LM (1975): Sprouting of seeds and nutritional composition of seeds and sprouts. J Food Sci 1975;40:552.
81. Wasserman BP, Montville TJ, Korwek EL (1988): Food biotechnology: a scientific status summary by the institute of food technologists' expert panel on food safety and nutrition. Food Tech 42(1):133–146.

Index

3